Natural Beauty recipe book

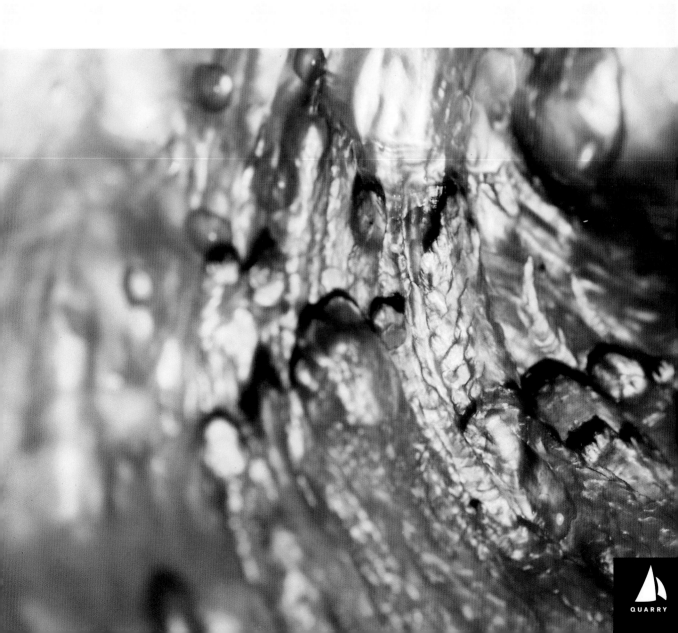

QUARRY

First published in the United States of America by
Quarry Books, a member of
Quayside Publishing Group
33 Commercial Street
Gloucester, Massachusetts 01930-5089
Telephone: (978) 282-9590
Fax: (978) 283-2742
www.rockpub.com

Library of Congress Cataloging-in-Publication Data available

ISBN 1-59253-298-5
ISBN-13: 978-1-59253-298-8

10 9 8 7 6 5 4 3 2 1

Design: Toby Matthews, toby.matthews@ntlworld.com
Photography: Robin Bath
Cover Design: Lori Wendin

Printed in Singapore

Grateful acknowledgment is given to Gill Farrer-Halls for her work from *How to Make Your Own Organic Cosmetics: Face Creams, Hair Rinses, and Body Lotions* (Quarry Books, 2004), pages 8–115; and for her work from *How to Make Your Own Organic Cosmetics: Soap and Scent* (Quarry Books, 2004), pages 116–221.

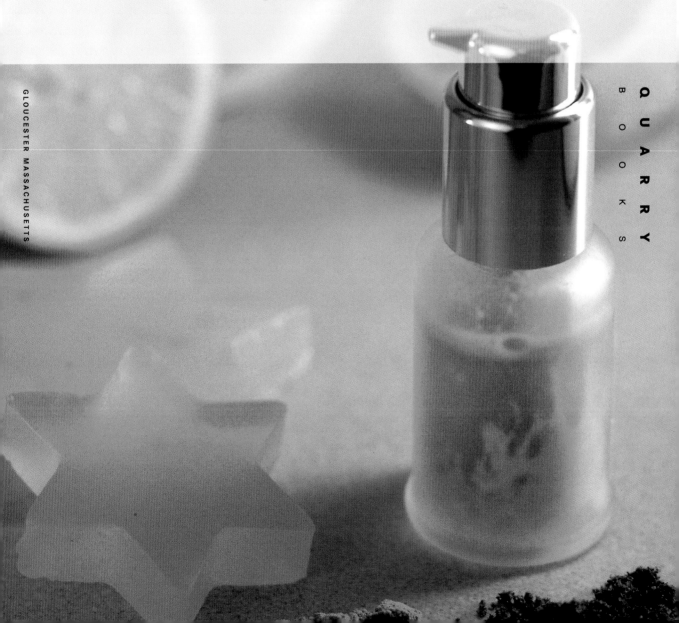

Natural Beauty recipe book

how to make your own organic cosmetics and beauty products

Gill Farrer-Halls

QUARRY BOOKS

GLOUCESTER MASSACHUSETTS

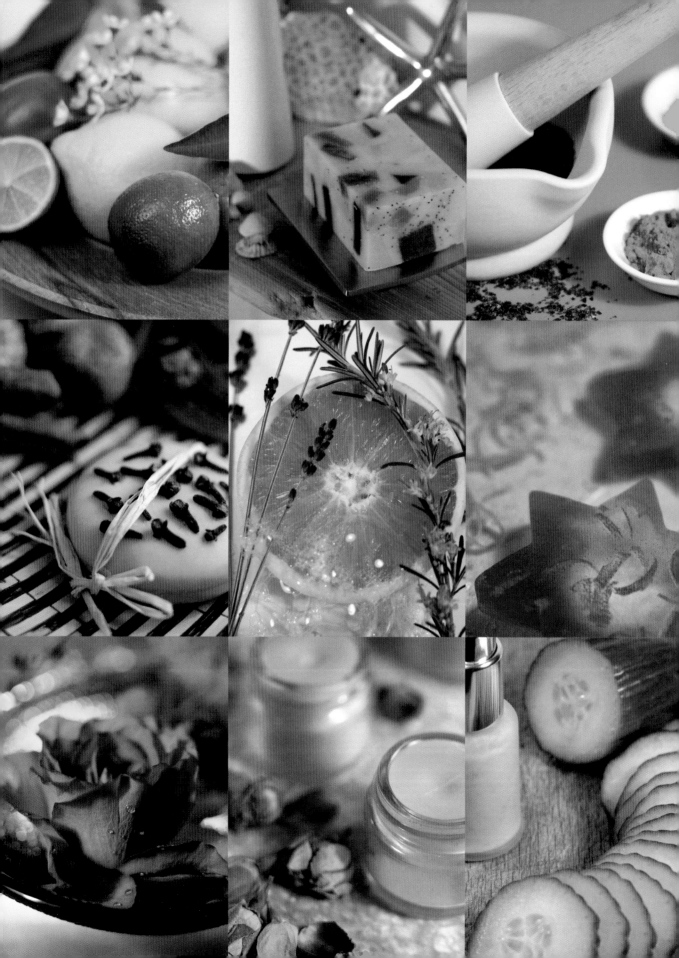

Contents

Introduction

Looking back over the last couple of decades, it is clear that increasing numbers of people have developed the desire for a more natural lifestyle. They have also realized the importance of an ethical responsibility and a considerate attitude toward the environment. These two concerns are united in the philosophy of organics. As part of the Green Movement, organics is seen as a positive counter force to the excessive use of chemicals in all aspects of our lives.

On hearing the word organic, most people usually think first of organic vegetables, fruits, and other natural foods, and then of how these foods are grown and produced. This in turn harks back to the traditional methods of local subsistence farming. This natural farming was practiced successfully until population growth and urbanization created a demand for large quantities of food to feed the populations of huge cities. Intensive farming methods were soon developed, and alongside the introduction of battery chickens and massive farm machinery came the use of agrochemicals.

Unfortunately, the use of agrochemicals such as herbicides, pesticides, and chemical fertilizers can cause long-term damage to the countryside and the birds and animals that inhabit it. Crops grown with agrochemicals do not taste as good, nor are they as full of natural goodness, as their organic counterparts. So, not only does organic agriculture mean growing natural produce without pesticides and herbicides but also ensuring that the environment is sustained healthily, and neither animals nor the countryside are exploited.

We are more than what we eat, however, and the organics philosophy can be extended beyond farming and food production into all other areas of life. We can respect ourselves and our whole environment by using natural, organic products wherever and whenever possible. Several companies manufacture biodegradable washing and cleaning products that do not pollute the environment. We can reuse plastic bags and compost our vegetable trimmings and leftover foods to minimize landfill sites. We can also recycle glass, paper, and aluminum cans; use natural, organic cosmetics; and wear clothes made of natural fibers.

In this spirit, *Natural Beauty Recipe Book* introduces the idea of making soaps and scents using natural, organic ingredients. Many products and ingredients in this book can be sourced from organic suppliers, and the recipes suggest using only vegetable and mineral ingredients that are not tested on animals. While obviously not designed for internal consumption, these soaps and scents are literally good enough to eat. Making and using these natural, organic soaps and scents is not only fun and creative, but good for you, body and spirit, and of benefit to the whole environment.

Many of the included ingredients and techniques for making cosmetics have been in use for thousands of years. They are known from long experience to be effective, safe, and beneficial to your skin. Some of the more modern, store-bought concoctions tend to use chemicals as well as animal and mineral substances. Not all of these substances are harmless to us, to animals, or to our environment. Therefore, the recipes here suggest using only organic and plant-based ingredients. When buying base lotions and creams, you can check whether these are made using organic plant-based ingredients.

The skin is far more important than just the wrapping around our body. It is, in fact, the body's largest organ, and it plays several roles in the healthy functioning of the whole body. One of the skin's major characteristics is that it is semipermeable. This means that certain substances can pass through the skin while others are simultaneously blocked. Hence, the skin both nourishes and protects the body. To illustrate, many toxins are sweated out through the skin and many nutrients are absorbed into the body through the skin. Bacteria are prevented entry to the body, and valuable bodily fluids are contained.

This knowledge emphasizes that what you put on your face and skin is as important as what you eat. Or, in other words, natural, organic cosmetics are as good for you as natural, organic foods. Some of the ingredients used to make your own cosmetics can be found in the kitchen, so—theoretically of course!—some of your homemade products are good enough to eat. Other ingredients can be sourced from organic cosmetics suppliers. The recipes in this book use only plant-based ingredients that are not tested on animals, so in keeping with the organics philosophy, you can have beauty without cruelty.

Effective skin care is necessary to keep the skin supple and in good condition so that it both looks beautiful and fulfills its functions. Using natural, organic substances such as flower waters, essential oils, honey, fruits, and so forth in homemade cosmetics can provide a wide range of skin treatments for all the different types of skin. The recipes included here range from simple additions to base creams and lotions to actually cooking up your own face and hand creams. No matter which recipes appeal to you, you can trust that your own homemade lotions and potions are natural and healthy. They also tend to work to be out cheaper than store-bought cosmetics, so you can afford to experiment and try out new skin care ideas.

In addition to recipes for face and hand creams and body lotions there are also recipes for making shampoos, conditioners, and rejuvenating hair treatments, as well as lip balms, skin toners, deodorants, aftershaves, and face masks—a comprehensive range of natural cosmetics to make, use, and enjoy.

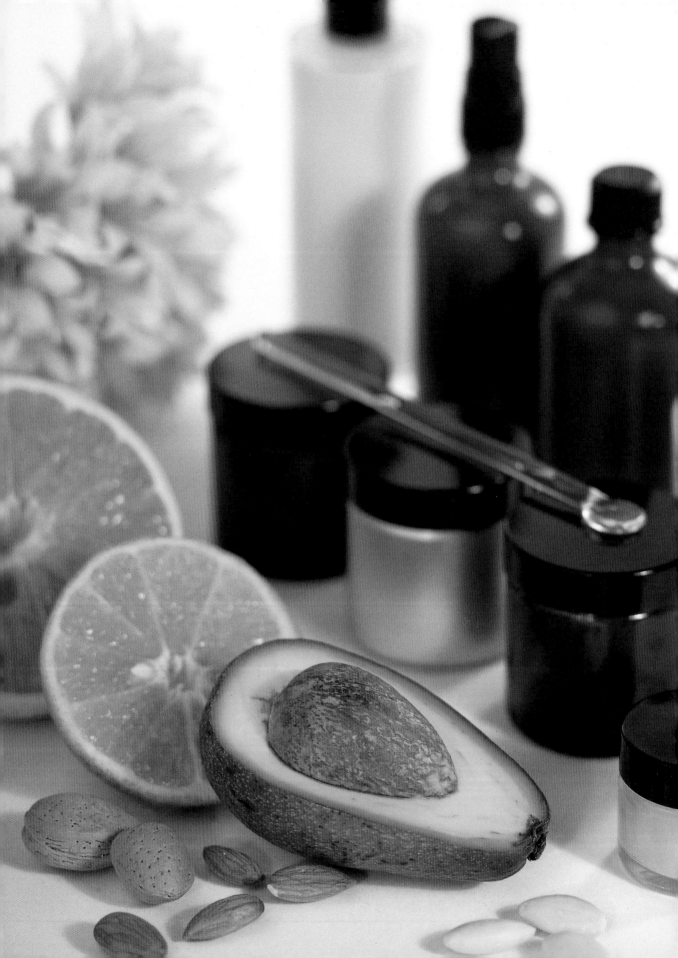

Chapter 1
Ingredients and Equipment

"Common sense and caution should go hand in hand when deciding on the choice of oils and strength of dilution."
—Patricia Davis, *author and aromatherapist*

Essential Oils and How to Use Them Safely

Essential oils are used extensively in the hand-made cosmetics in this book. The oils bring healing and protective skin-care qualities to all the products, as well as enhancing these products with their delightful fragrances. Essential oils are highly concentrated, as can be seen by the fact that it takes thousands of jasmine petals to produce a single drop of jasmine. This potency must be respected, and thus how you handle essential oils is important. Because essential oils are powerful and concentrated, they can be toxic if used incorrectly. However, if you handle oils carefully and follow these simple guidelines, they are quite safe for all your homemade cosmetics.

• Never take essential oils orally. It is illegal for even a qualified aromatherapist to suggest this. Avoid all contact with the mouth and eyes.

• Some essential oils can cause skin irritation if they are applied undiluted to the skin, therefore this is not recommended. Apply only properly diluted essential oils to the skin.

• The A–Z of Essential Oils section on page 12 indicates which oils might cause skin irritation for those with sensitive skin. Occasionally, a slight redness or itchiness might occur from using these or any other essential oil. If this happens, apply some base cream or base oil, such as almond oil, to the affected area and place a cold, wet cloth on the affected area until the redness or itchiness disappears.

• Do not be tempted to increase the amount of essential oils used in the recipes and follow the instructions carefully.

• If you accidentally splash a drop of essential oil in your eye, use a small amount of base oil to dilute the essential oil, absorb this with a soft cloth, then rinse the eyes with cold water.

• A few essential oils, such as bergamot, lemon, and the other citrus oils, are phototoxic. This means they might cause skin discoloration when exposed to bright sunlight, though once incorporated into skin-care products they are diluted and quite safe. However, it is best to avoid using face creams and body lotions containing bergamot and other citrus oils if the weather is hot and sunny.

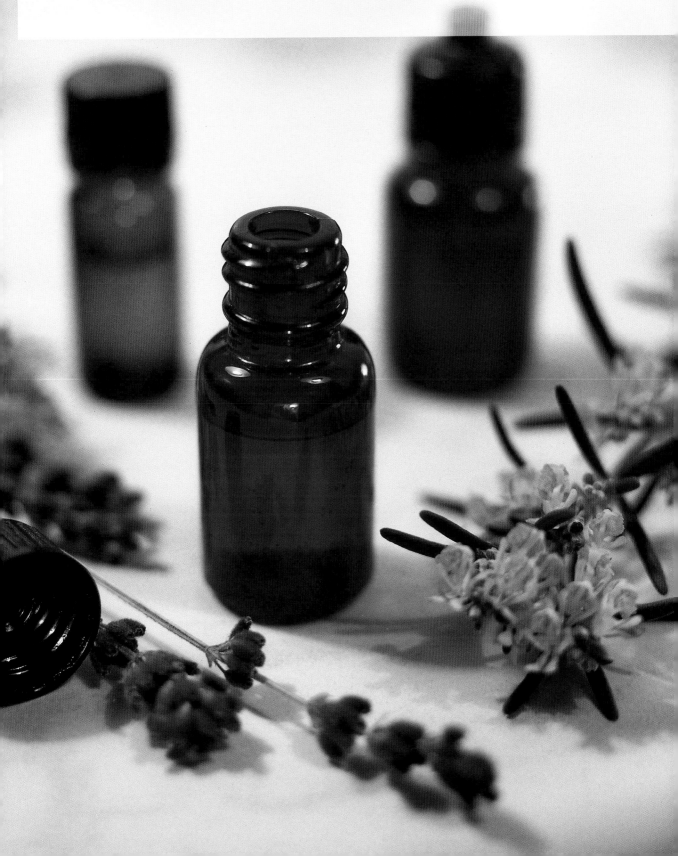

Tip: When you finish an essential oil and the bottle is empty, reward yourself with a beaufully fragranced, relaxing bath by rinsing it out in the water.

A–Z of Essential Oils

Essential oils are nature's gift. They are distilled from the naturally occurring essences in aromatic plants. Many essential oils are distilled from organically grown plants, and these are the best to use in making your cosmetics. Below is a list of the main essential oils used in the recipes, together with a description of their fragrances and qualities. A "P" indicates the oil should not to be used during pregnancy. An "S" indicates a possibility of skin irritation for people with sensitive skin.

Basil/Holy Basil (ocimum basilicum/sanctum)
Basil is a familiar culinary herb. The essential oil has sweet, green, herbaceous top notes and spicy, liquorice undertones. Holy basil has a similar aroma, but with more depth. P

Bergamot (citrus bergamia)
Bergamot is grown in Italy, and is the finest of the citrus oils. It has fresh, lemon, top notes and floral, balsamic undertones. S

Chamomile Roman/Chamomile German
(anthemis nobilis/matricaria chamomilla)
Chamomile has a calming, soothing effect on the skin. The fragrance has hints of apple among bitter, herbaceous undertones and warm, flowery top notes. P

Frankincense (boswellia carteri)
Frankincense was used in the embalming of bodies in ancient Egypt, and has antiaging properties. It combines citrus, turpentine top notes with undertones of camphor and balsamic wood smoke.

Geranium (pelargonium gravolens)
Geranium helps regulate sebum production in the skin and is generally balancing. It has light, green top notes and soft, rosy, floral undertones. P

Ginger (zingiber officinalis)
Ginger is used in cooking and teas as a stimulating, fortifying digestive. The essential oil has sharp, green top notes and fiery, woody, sweet, spicy undertones. S

Jasmine (jasminum officinale)
Jasmine combines a powerful, heady fragrance with excellent skin care properties, especially for dry, sensitive skin. Jasmine has sweet, floral, exotic top notes and heady, warm, honeyed undertones. P

Lavender (lavandula vera)
Lavender is the most popular and widely used essential oil, and has soothing, anti-inflammatory properties. Lavender's calming qualities help promote sleep. It has clean, fresh, floral top notes and subtle, green, herbaceous undertones.

Lemon (citrus limon)
The fresh smell of lemon is a familiar one. Lemon is also an astringent, making it useful for greasy skin. Lemon has clean, fresh, light, sharp top notes with slightly sweet, citrus undertones. S

Neroli/Orange Blossom (citrus bigardia/aurantium)
Traditionally used in wedding bouquets, neroli calms and soothes the skin. The delightful fragrance has delicate, fresh, floral top notes and warm, heady, bittersweet undertones.

Orange (citrus sinensis)
This essential oil is distilled from the sweet orange variety. Orange shares some of the properties of neroli, and works well in skin toners and deodorants. It has sweet, fresh, fruity top notes and radiant, sensuous undertones.

Palmarosa (cymbopogon martinii)
This is a delicate, gentle essential oil distilled from a grass closely related to lemongrass. Palmarosa has sweet, light, floral top notes with subtle lemon and geranium undertones.

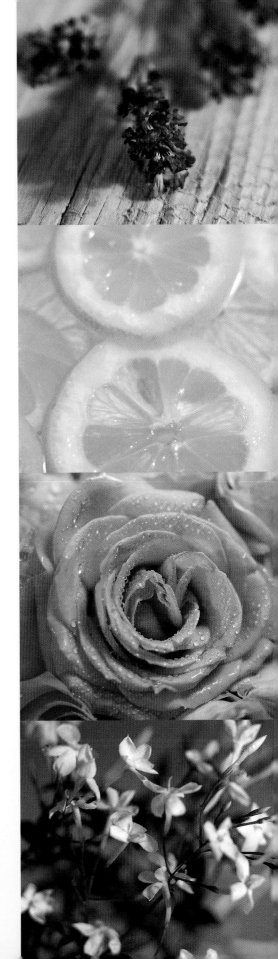

Petitgrain (citrus aurantium)

The refreshing aroma of petitgrain is often used in skin care products, and it has a relaxing, balancing quality. Petitgrain shares many of the qualities of neroli, and has fresh, floral, citrus top notes and light, woody undertones.

Rose (rosa centifolia/damascena)

Romantic rose has often been described as the queen of flowers, and it is best of all oils in skin care preparations. Rose has deep, sweet, floral top notes with dusky, honeyed undertones. P

Rosemary (rosmarinus officinalis)

"Rosemary for remembrance" is a folk saying, and rosemary is a mental stimulant. Rosemary has sharp, fresh, green, top notes and herbaceous, camphoraceous undertones. P

Rosewood (aniba rosaeodora)

Rosewood is an endangered species, so make sure the oil you buy comes from a sustainable rosewood plantation. Rosewood is both subtle and powerful with soft, floral top notes and sweet, woody undertones.

Sandalwood (santalum album)

Sandalwood's warm, heavy fragrance increases over time, and it is beneficial for all skin types. Sandalwood has sweet, woody, roselike top notes and deep, balsamic, spicy, oriental undertones.

Ylang Ylang (cananga odorata)

Ylang ylang is much used in the cosmetics industry for its voluptuous, exotic fragrance. It has intensely sweet, almond, floral, tropical top notes and slightly cloying, creamy, spicy undertones.

Equipment, Ingredients, and Containers

Equipment and Containers

Most of the equipment—and some of the ingredients—you need to make skin-care products can be found in the kitchen. A glass stirring rod is recommended, and can be purchased from one of the specialist suppliers listed on pages 222–223 or from a kitchen-supply store. You will also need to purchase a variety of glass jars in a range of different sizes, as these will be the containers for your skin creams, cleansers, and lip balms. Dark glass bottles, some with spray attachments and others with caps, are required for skin toners, body lotions, and deodorants.

Ingredients

All the ingredients below can be purchased from the specialist suppliers listed on pages 222–223, although some of these ingredients may also be found in your local natural-health store. Here are the main ingredients you will need to make your own cosmetics.

- Base products: skin lotion, cleanser, and cream, and hair shampoo and conditioner

- A range of essential oils, herbal tinctures, and flower waters

- Base oils: almond, apricot, rosehip seed, kukui nut, calendula, carrot, vitamin E, evening primrose, jojoba, avocado

- Beeswax, shea butter, Monoi de Tahiti, and cocoa butter

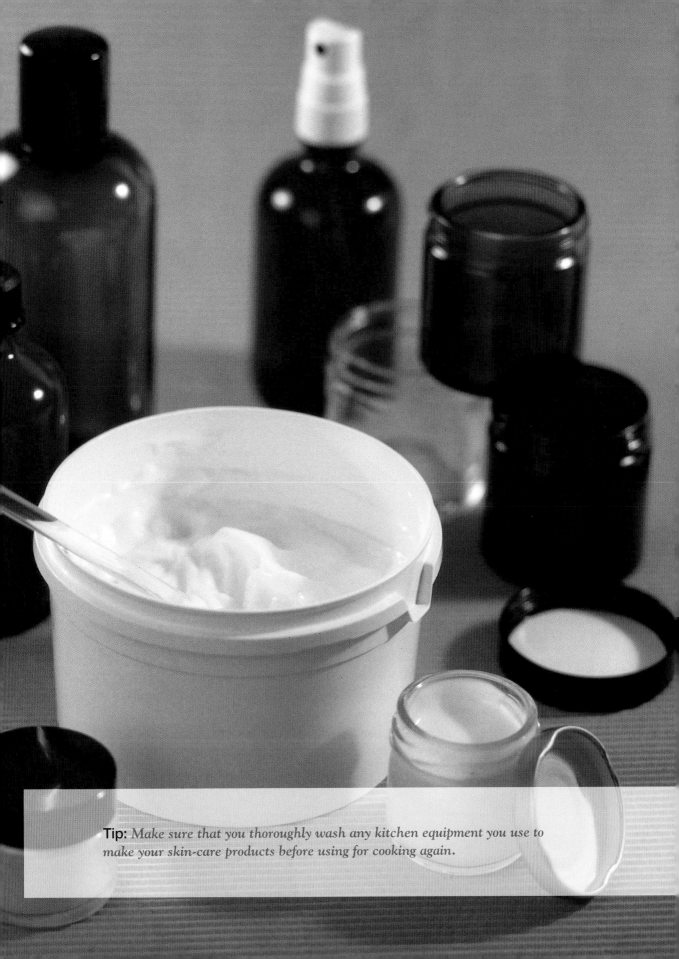

Tip: *Make sure that you thoroughly wash any kitchen equipment you use to make your skin-care products before using for cooking again.*

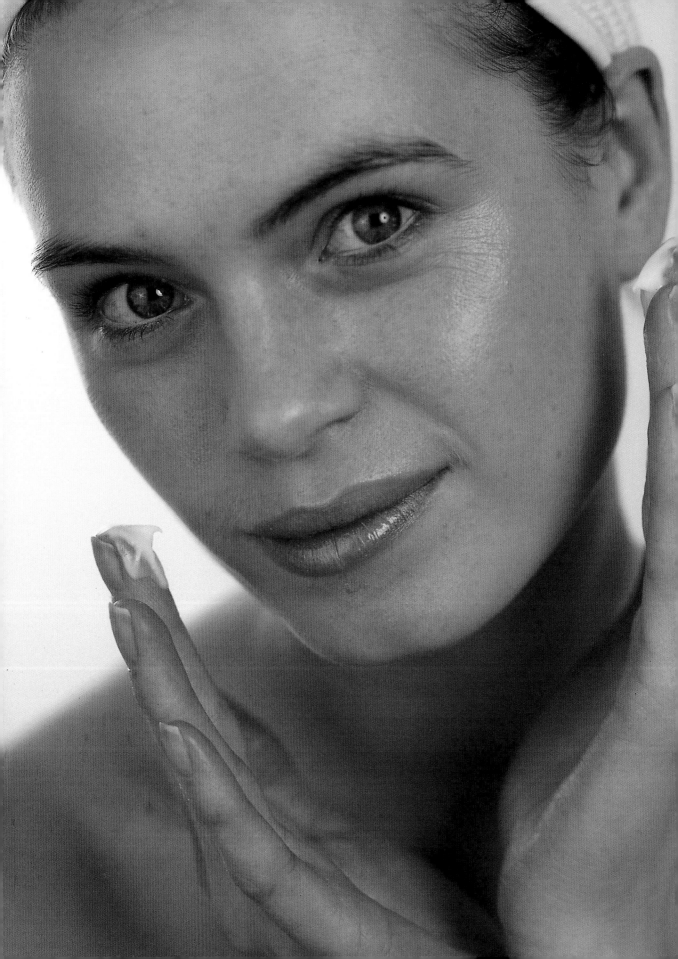

Chapter 2

Quick and Easy Everyday Face Products

"The beauty of base products derives from simplicity; they are especially mild, gentle, and pure, making them great to use."

–Baldwins catalog

Creating Your Own Skin Care Cosmetics

The recipes in this chapter are quick and simple to make, so you can easily get started creating your own cosmetics. These recipes also provide a selection of daily cleansing, toning, and moisturizing products. They offer ideas for different additions to the base cleansers, toners, and moisturizers, so you can personalize all your face care products to suit your skin. By following a few easy, step-by-step instructions you can transform your daily face care regime.

You probably already know your skin type, and therefore which face care products are suitable for your face. However, it is a good idea to check the condition of your skin. Seasonal factors, such as turning on the central heating or spending time in the sun, affect the skin. Differences in temperature, whether the climate is damp or dry, and how much wind you are exposed to all affect the condition of your skin and especially your face. Therefore, several different kinds of cleansers, toners, and moisturizers can all have their uses at different times throughout the year.

You should also consider other factors that affect your skin, such as whether your general health is good and what types of food you eat. Taking a holistic approach to caring for your skin helps ensure you face the world looking as good as possible. This means looking at what you eat and making changes to help your skin from within. Some people can eat cream cakes and chips and still have a beautiful figure and lovely skin, but

they are in a tiny minority. Most of us need to eat sensibly to keep our bodies and our skin in good condition.

Alongside making your own daily face care products, you can make a few dietary changes. It is important to drink a lot of spring water. This flushes toxins out of the body through the urinary system, which means they don't have to be expelled through the skin. Reducing salt and caffeine and drinking herbal tea also helps. Eating less fried and processed foods, sugar, and red meat while increasing your consumption of organic fresh fruit and vegetables and whole grains can help bring a healthy glow to your face.

Another lifestyle factor that affects the skin is exercise. If you work in an office, the chances are you spend little time outside. Taking a daily walk in the park and escaping to the countryside is beneficial. This reduces exposure to air pollution and increases your intake of fresh air. Exercise generally stimulates the circulation and increases blood flow, which sends nutrients through the blood to nourish all parts of the body.

Making and using your own quick and easy daily face products, together with a few lifestyle changes, can improve the appearance of your face within a couple of weeks—all without expending too much time and effort. Caring for your face in this holistic way not only makes you look good but helps you feel healthy too.

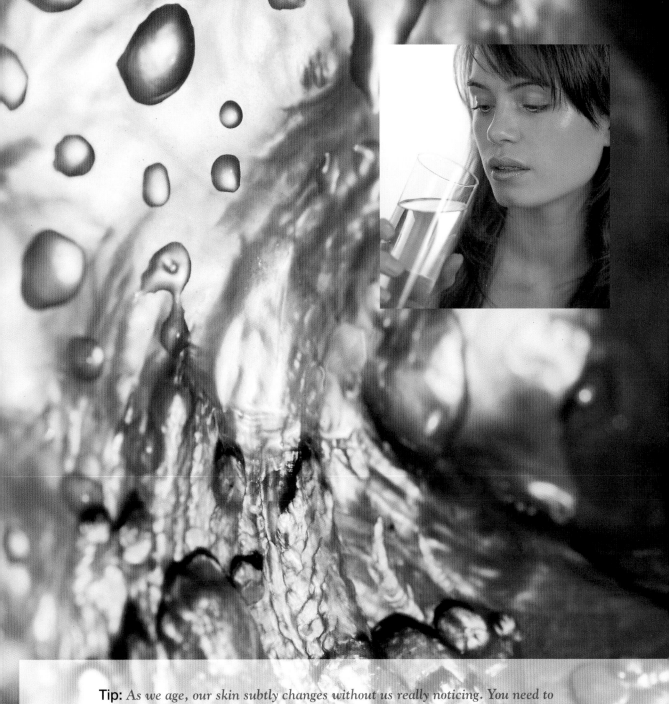

Tip: *As we age, our skin subtly changes without us really noticing. You need to take this into account by checking the condition of your skin before choosing your skin-care products and being prepared to modify your choice accordingly.*

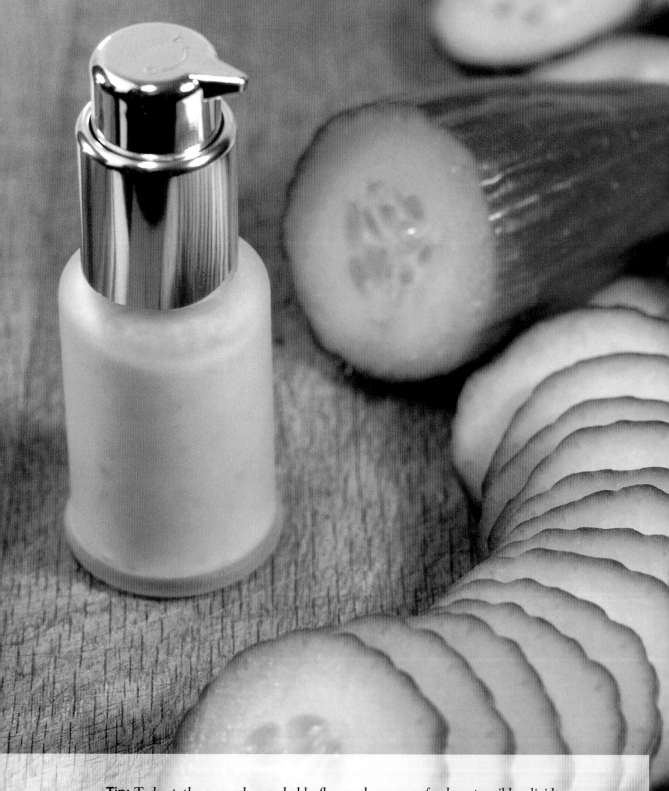

Tip: *To keep the cucumber and elderflower cleanser as fresh as possible, divide the amount you make into two portions. Pour one part into a bottle for current use and pour the other portion into another bottle that you can keep in the refrigerator until you are ready to use it.*

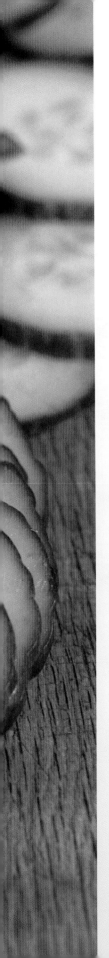

Face Cleansers

Cleansing the skin properly, especially the face, is fundamental to good skin care. This is even more important if you live in a city or near an industrial area, as airborne toxins will readily adhere to your face, causing damage and premature aging.

Cleansing is the first of the three step, twice daily face care regime of cleansing, toning, and moisturizing. Because facial skin is so delicate, soap is much too harsh and drying to use to wash the face.

Special face cleansers, mostly based around a cream or a lotion, are the best way to cleanse your face thoroughly yet gently. The following cleansers use a cleansing lotion base, and are best applied and wiped off with damp cotton balls.

Creamy Cucumber and Elderflower

Cucumber features in many commercial face cleansers, as it is a tried and trusted natural astringent and cleansing agent. Here, we use organic cucumber to create a fresh, natural cleanser, suitable for all skin types. Elder-flowers are healing and astringent.

what's in it?
5 oz (150 ml) cleansing lotion base
⅓ of a fresh, organic cucumber
7 drops elderflower tincture
5 drops lemon essential oil

how's it made?
1 Wash the cucumber thoroughly in cold water. Chop a third of the cucumber roughly, place it in a blender, and puree.

2 Strain the cucumber through a piece of clean muslin. Squeeze the cloth to extract the juice.

3 Measure the cleansing lotion base into a glass container with a good pouring spout. Add the cucumber juice and stir thoroughly. Add the elderflower tincture and lemon oil and stir to thoroughly combine all the ingredients.

4 Pour the mixture into two bottles. Label them clearly. One is ready for use and the other can be stored in the refrigerator for up to one month.

Palmarosa and Linden Blossom

The fresh, clean smell of palmarosa blends beautifully with the sweet, slightly honeyed tones of linden flower water to create a delicate, fragrant cleanser, suitable for all skin types. Palmarosa is astringent, helps balance sebum production, and is reputed to help smooth out wrinkles.

what's in it?

5 oz (150 ml) cleansing lotion base

1 tbsp (15 ml) linden flower water

30 drops palmarosa

how's it made?

1 Measure the cleansing lotion base into a glass container with a good pouring spout.

2 Add the linden flower water and mix thoroughly. This will create a lotion rather than a cream. You could add a little less or a little more flower water according to preference.

3 Add the drops of palmarosa carefully, and stir well to incorporate thoroughly into the mixture.

4 Pour into a bottle and label. The cleanser is ready to use.

Mild Meadowsweet

Meadowsweet is anti-inflammatory and astringent, and makes a useful addition to this cleanser. Meadowsweet is also mildly analgesic because it contains salicylic acid—nature's own natural aspirin. The addition of rose flower water and neroli make this gentle, sweet smelling cleanser especially mild and suited to sensitive, inflamed, or irritated skin.

what's in it?

5 oz (150 ml) cleansing lotion base

10 drops meadowsweet tincture

1 tbsp (15 ml) rose flower water

20 drops neroli

how's it made?

1 Measure the cleansing lotion base into a glass container with a good pouring spout.

2 Add the rose flower water and mix thoroughly. This will create a lotion rather than a cream. You could add a little less or a little more flower water according to preference.

3 Add the drops of neroli and meadowsweet carefully, and stir well to incorporate thoroughly into the mixture.

4 Pour into a bottle and label. The cleanser is ready to use.

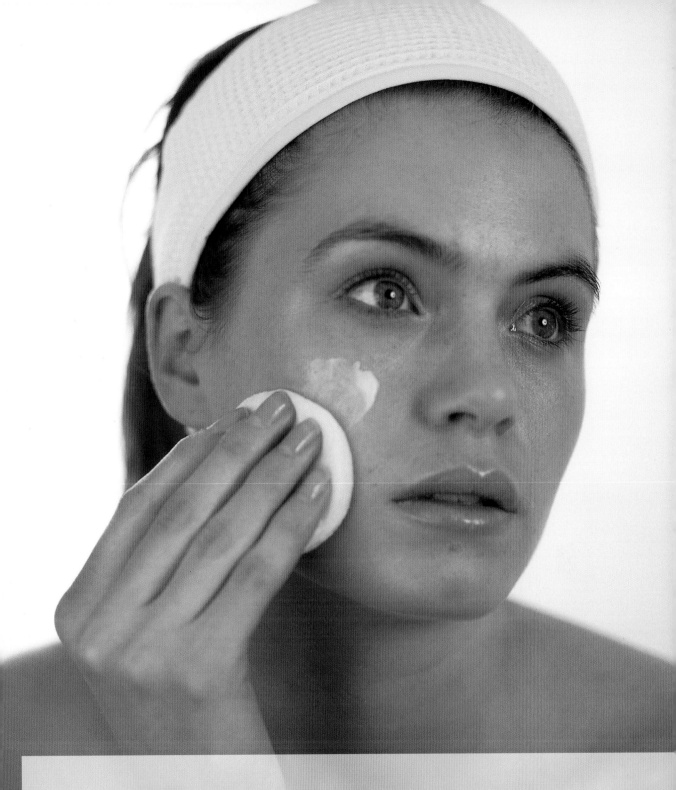

Did You Know? *Palmarosa is one of a few essential oils that helps keep the skin clear and fresh by stimulating healthy cellular regeneration.*

Tip: *Eyebright also helps eyes that have a tendency for weepiness caused by sensitivity to light, so this is a good eye cleanser if your eyes are light sensitive.*

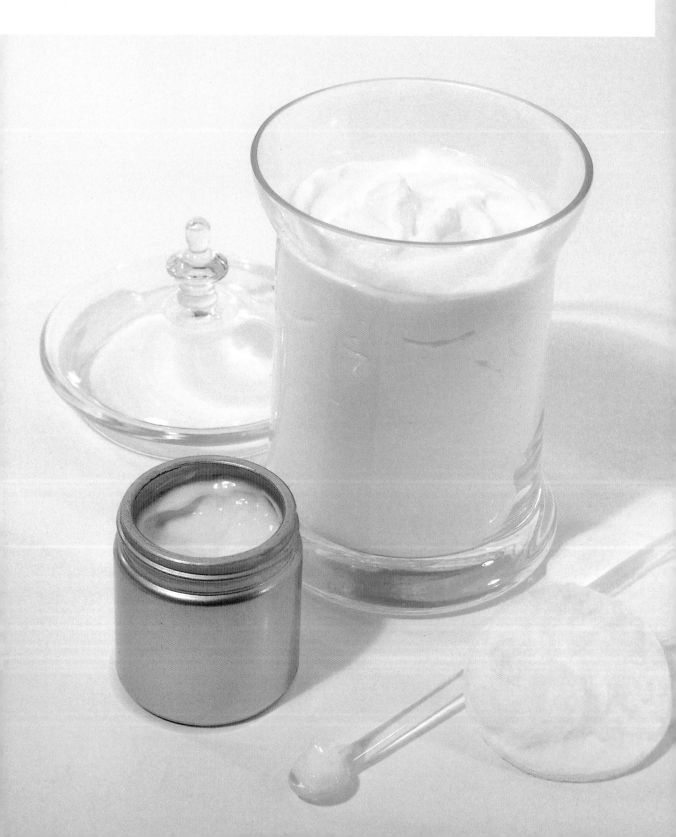

Eye Area Cleansers

The delicate skin around the eyes needs extra special care and attention. Some commercial cleansers contain harsh ingredients or a high percentage of alcohol, which are quite unsuitable for the delicate area around the eyes. The following two cleansers contain gentle oils, flower waters, and herbal tinctures that are especially suited to gently cleansing the eye area.

However, as with all face care products, care must be taken not to get any of the eye cleanser into the eyes themselves.

If you accidentally rub a little cleanser into your eyes, simply rinse out with cold water and pat the eyes dry. Use damp cotton balls to apply and wipe off the eye area cleansers.

Gentle Eyebright

As the name suggests, eyebright is a herb that has a special affinity with the eyes. It is especially helpful if there is any inflammation or stinging around the eyes. In this cleanser, tincture of eyebright is mixed with an infusion of chamomile to create a gentle cleanser suitable for the eye area, especially if the eyes are red and tired.

what's in it?
2 tbsp (25 ml) cleansing lotion base
2 drops eyebright tincture
1 tsp (5 ml) chamomile infusion (see step 3)

how's it made?

1 Measure the cleansing lotion base into a 2 oz (50 ml) glass jar.

2 Add the eyebright tincture to the base lotion. Mix thoroughly.

3 Make an infusion of chamomile by steeping one organic chamomile tea bag for ten minutes. Let cool and stir 1 tsp (5 ml) of the infusion thoroughly into the eye cleanser.

4 Pour the cleanser into a jar and label it. The eye area cleanser is ready to use.

Evening Primrose and Cornflower Water

Evening primrose oil is rich in gamma linoleic acid, an essential fatty acid. It has been shown to help psoriasis, eczema, and other skin conditions, and is generally useful for sensitive, delicate skin. The clean, fresh scent of cornflower water also lightly fragrances this eye area cleanser.

what's in it?

2 tbsp (25 ml) cleansing lotion base
1 evening primrose oil capsule
1 tsp (5 ml) cornflower water

how's it made?

1 Measure the cleansing lotion base into a 2 oz (50 ml) glass jar.

2 Pierce the capsule of evening primrose oil with a pin and squeeze out the oil into the base lotion. Mix thoroughly.

3 Add the cornflower water to the mixture and stir thoroughly.

4 Pour the cleanser into a jar and label it. The eye area cleanser is ready to use.

Tip: *Cornflower water has traditionally been used to soothe tired eyes, help eye infections, and provide general care for the eye area.*

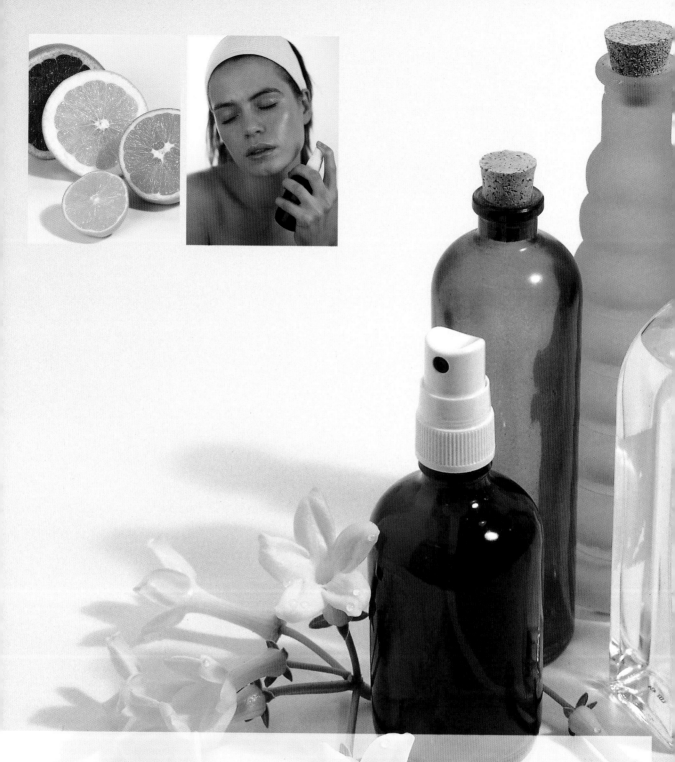

Did You Know? *Orange flower water is obtained by distillation of orange blossom petals. This distillation process is actually undertaken to produce the essential oil neroli. The orange flower water is considered a by-product of this process, although it is valuable in its own right. Using products containing both neroli and orange flower water utilizes the synergy of the whole plant.*

Toners

Skin toners are used to tighten the skin's pores after cleansing. Toners also function to remove traces of cleanser, so they are a valuable part of a skin care regime. However, many store-bought toners contain harsh ingredients that dry the skin, leaving your face feeling dry and tight.

Making your own skin toners is a simple process, and well worth the effort. By using some of the recipes that follow, you can be sure you are using only pure, natural, and organic ingredients that are kind and gentle to your skin and of benefit to your complexion.

Fresh and Fruity

This fresh smelling skin toner is a treat to use in the morning, as the fragrance is uplifting and invigorating. This astringent toner is ideal for youthful and oily skins, though it is gentle enough for all skin types. The addition of citrus essential oils helps tone the complexion, and leaves your skin feeling clean and refreshed.

what's in it?

1 tbsp (10 ml) high proof vodka

2 drops grapefruit

2 drops neroli

2 drops orange

2 drops lemon

2 tbsp (25 ml) witch hazel

1 cup (250 ml) orange flower water

how's it made?

1 Pour the high proof vodka into a clean, dry glass bottle large enough to hold at least 11 oz (300 ml) of liquid. You can use a spray bottle to easily apply the toner.

2 Add the essential oils to the vodka and shake vigorously to dissolve the oils.

3 Add the witch hazel and shake well, followed by the orange flower water. Shake the bottle until all the ingredients have blended together well.

4 The skin toner is ready to use. However, the essential oils will separate slightly over time, so shake the bottle just before using each time.

Rose and Geranium Toner

This skin toner is suited to all skin types, as the main action of the essential oils is balancing. However, rose is also especially suited to dry and mature skin. The deep, honeyed aroma of roses from both rose essential oil and from the rose water mingles with the fresh, floral scent of geranium to make a delightful, delicate skin toner.

what's in it?

1 tbsp (10 ml) high proof vodka
4 drops rose
4 drops geranium
2 tbsp (25 ml) witch hazel
1 cup (250 ml) rose flower water

how's it made?

1 Pour the high proof vodka into a clean, dry glass bottle large enough to hold at least 11 oz (300 ml) of liquid. You can use a spray bottle to easily apply the toner.

2 Add the essential oils to the vodka and shake vigorously to dissolve the oils.

3 Add the witch hazel and shake well, followed by the rose flower water. Shake the bottle until all the ingredients have blended together well.

4 The skin toner is ready to use. However, the essential oils will separate slightly over time, so shake the bottle just before using each time.

Orange Flower Blossom and Petitgrain

The fresh, woody smell of petitgrain in this skin toner is complemented by the sweet, delicate scent of neroli. The gentle action of linden flower water makes this toner suitable for all skin types, but it is especially great for dry and sensitive skin. The sweet, honeyed fragrance of linden blossom blends with palmarosa and chamomile to give a balanced overall fragrance.

what's in it?

1 tbsp (10 ml) high proof vodka
2 drops neroli
2 drops petitgrain
2 drops chamomile
2 drops palmarosa
2 tbsp (25 ml) witch hazel
1 cup (250 ml) linden flower water

how's it made?

1 Pour the high proof vodka into a clean, dry glass bottle large enough to hold at least 11 oz (300 ml) of liquid. You can use a spray bottle to easily apply the toner.

2 Add the essential oils to the vodka and shake vigorously to dissolve the oils.

3 Add the witch hazel and shake well, followed by the linden flower water. Shake the bottle until all the ingredients have blended together well.

4 The skin toner is ready to use. However, the essential oils will separate slightly over time, so shake the bottle just before using each time.

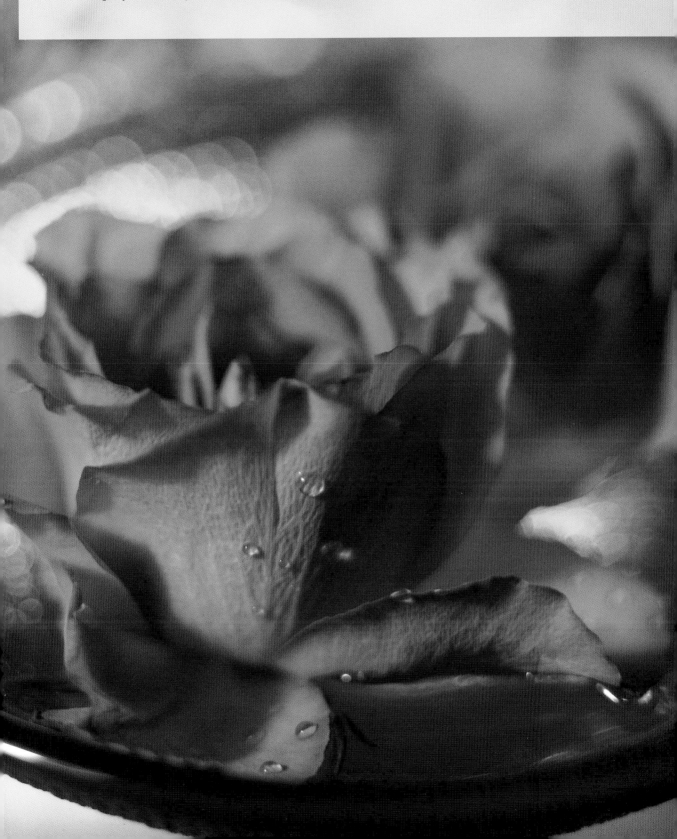

Did You Know? *Skin toners are wonderfully cooling and refreshing when sprayed on the face on a hot, sunny day.*

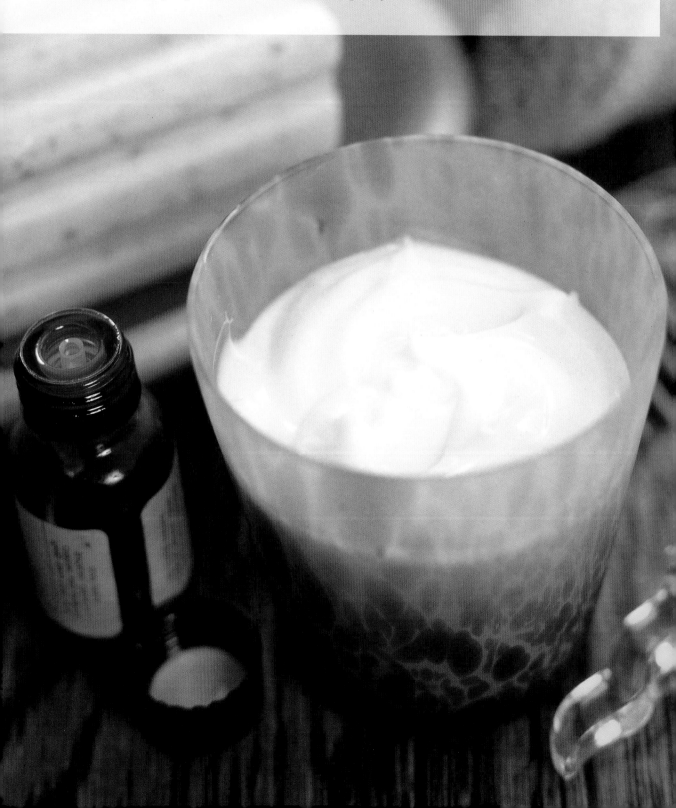

Did You Know? *The extensive reputation of sandalwood as a perfume is partly due to its fragrance, which appeals to both women and men. However, sandalwood's sweet, woody perfume is reputed to be an aphrodisiac, and its popularity is perhaps a testament to this quality.*

Moisturizing Creams

In many ways, moisturizers are the most important product throughout the whole skin-care range. They nourish, hydrate, and protect the skin, and keep it supple and able to fulfill its functions for the body.

If you were stuck on a desert island and could take only one skin-care product with you, it would have to be a good, basic moisturizer.

The moisturizer recipes here are really quick and simple to make. Before starting, you need to buy a cream base from a reputable supplier (see pages 222–223). Most suppliers offer at least two cream bases—a light one and a richer, heavier one. This will give you a lighter day moisturizer and a richer night cream. Choose the cream that suits your skin best, or make up different moisturizers by combining both types.

Kukui Nut and Sandalwood

Kukui nut oil is high in linoleic and linolenic fatty acids, which are essential for healthy skin. Kukui nut oil is also easily absorbed by the skin and is known to benefit acne, eczema, and psoriasis. Sandalwood is much used in skin care and is beneficial for all skin types, especially helping oily skin as it is slightly astringent. This cream is suited to all skin types and both sexes, so it makes a good general moisturizer for everyone in the family.

what's in it?
2 tbsp (30 gm) of your chosen cream base

1 tsp (2 ml) kukui nut oil

12 drops sandalwood

how's it made?
1 Half fill a clean glass jar (either a 2 or 2½ oz [50 or 60 gm] size) with your chosen cream base.

2 Stir in the kukui nut oil using a glass stirring rod or a chopstick. Make sure the oil is thoroughly blended into the cream.

3 Carefully add the sandalwood. Stir in thoroughly, making sure the essential oil is completely dispersed throughout the cream. The cream is now ready to use.

Calendula and Neroli

The addition of macerated calendula oil gives this cream healing and anti-inflammatory properties, and it soothes and softens the skin. Neroli essential oil gives a delicate, sweet scent. Neroli is calming and good for nerves, and it soothes sensitive, delicate skin. Neroli also helps in the regeneration of new skin cells, which keeps the skin looking fresh and smooth. This moisturizer is particularly suited to dry, sensitive skin, and for sore or chapped skin, redness, or broken thread veins.

what's in it?

2 tbsp (30 gm) of your chosen cream base

1 tsp (3 ml) macerated calendula oil

10 drops neroli

how's it made?

1 Half fill a clean glass jar (either a 2 or 2½ oz [50 or 60 gm] size) with your chosen cream base.

2 Stir in the calendula oil using a glass stirring rod or a chopstick. Make sure the oil is thoroughly blended into the cream.

3 Carefully add the neroli. Stir in thoroughly, making sure the essential oil is thoroughly dispersed throughout the cream. The cream is ready to use.

Rosewood and Rose with Rosehip Seed Oil

The wonderful fragrance of rose is balanced with the woody, floral perfume of rosewood. Together they produce a delicate feminine perfume. Both these oils are excellent in face creams. Rosehip seed oil is rich in G.L.A. or gamma linoleic acid, which is valuable in treating a variety of skin problems, especially if there is inflammation. This cream is particularly suited to dry, sensitive, or mature skin, but makes a beautiful moisturizer for all skin types.

what's in it?

2 tbsp (30 gm) of your chosen cream base

1 tsp (3 ml) rosehip seed oil

4 drops rose

7 drops rosewood

how's it made?

1 Half fill a clean glass jar (either a 2 or 2½ oz [50 or 60 gm] size) with your chosen cream base.

2 Stir in the rosehip seed oil using a glass stirring rod or a chopstick. Make sure the oil is thoroughly blended into the cream.

3 Carefully add the rose and rosewood. Stir in thoroughly, making sure the essential oils are completely dispersed throughout the cream. The cream is ready to use.

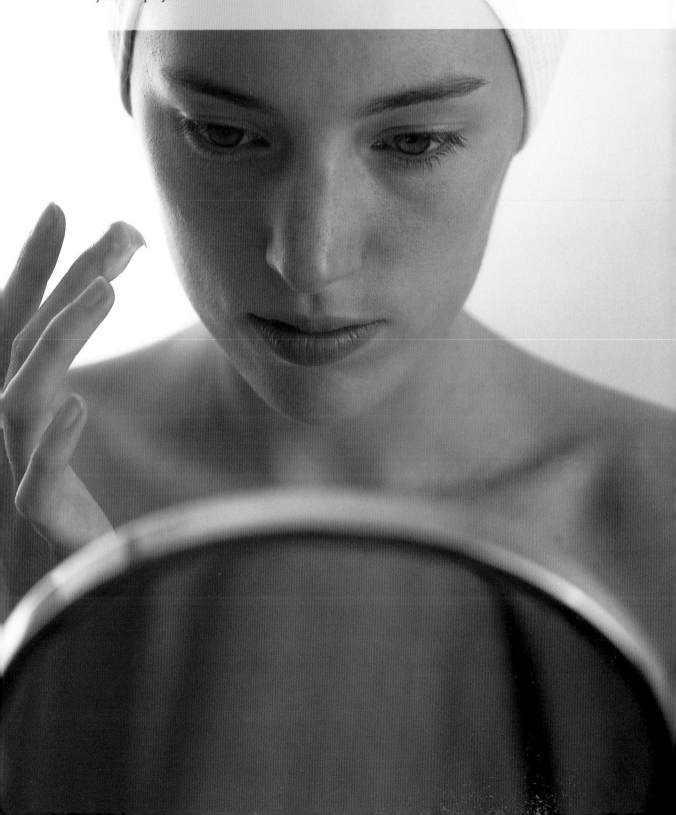

Did You Know? *Neroli is distilled from the flowers of the bitter orange, which has grown for centuries around Seville. This hauntingly beautiful fragranced essential oil is named after an Italian princess who used it as her favorite perfume.*

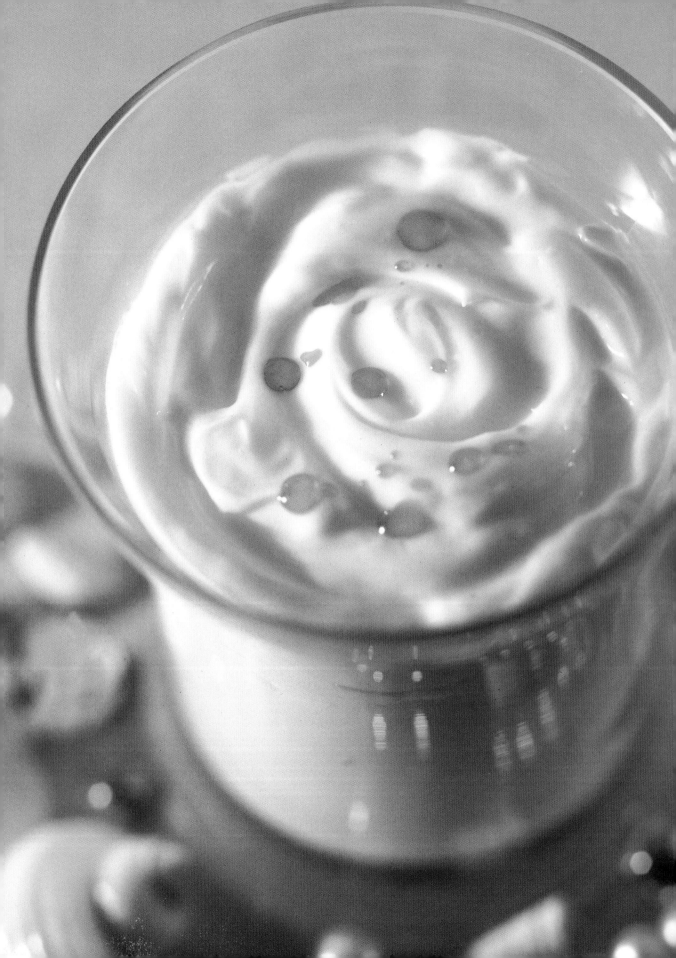

Chapter 3

Making Creams, Lotions, and Lip Balms

"Since essential oils are soluble in oil and alcohol and impart their scent to water, they provide the ideal ingredient for cosmetics and general skin care."

–Julia Lawless, *author and aromatherapist*

Homemade Face Creams

Making your own skin-care products can be very rewarding. Although it is fun to experiment with the wide range of commercial skin-care creams and lotions available these days, they are often expensive. In addition, you are probably not familiar with some of the ingredients the creams are made from, and many of these substances are inorganic and synthetic. If you develop a skin rash or allergy from using a store-bought cream, not only do you not know exactly what caused it but you have to throw away what was probably an expensive item.

Creating you own creams, lotions, and balms from scratch means you have the satisfaction of knowing every single ingredient that has gone into the making of the product. You can ensure that you use only pure, natural, plant-based constituents, and you can choose organic ingredients whenever possible. The chances of developing an allergic reaction to your own homemade face creams and body lotions are far less than if you use many of the store-bought skin-care products.

Incorporating essential oils for their skin-care properties enriches the creams and lotions, provides natural healing qualities, and imparts a natural fragrance. The wide range of essential oils available gives you the flexibility to make a variety of skin-care products for different skin types from a few basic formulas. In this way, you end up with high-quality, natural skin creams and lotions at a much cheaper cost than their commercial equivalents.

However, there is one minor drawback in making your own face creams. Commercial face-cream manufacturers use specialized equipment, including emulsifying machines. These help the fat-based ingredients and the water-based ingredients blend into the light, fluffy, homogenous face creams you usually purchase. Your homemade creams will not emulsify in quite the same way.

This means you will end up with quite oily creams in some instances, as not all the fat-based ingredients will emulsify fully with the water-based ingredients. This doesn't make the cream any less effective, but it does take longer for it to absorb into the skin. This can be ideal; for example gardeners or manual workers, who often have very dry, cracked skin, will enjoy the hand creams as their skin will readily absorb these rich creams.

The best thing to do is to experiment. If you find any of your homemade face or hand creams too rich, or they take too long to absorb into your skin, mix them into a cream base. Try half and half to start with, and adjust the proportion of cream base to homemade cream to get exactly the texture that suits your skin best. With a bit of experimentation, you will end up with a selection of natural, beautifully fragranced skin creams that suit your own individual skin type and condition.

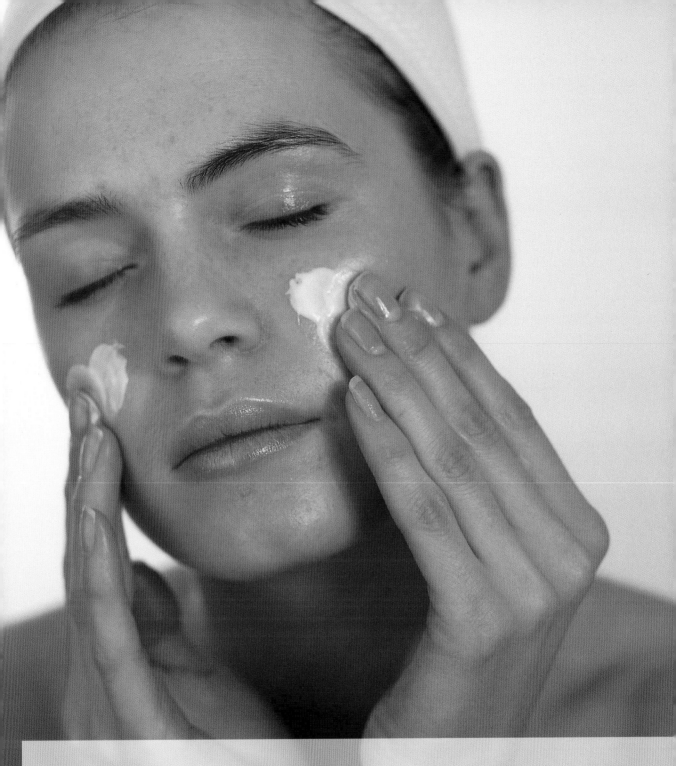

Tip: In some recipes, liquids are measured by volume and in others they are measured by weight. This makes no difference to the creams; it's simply how the different recipes were originally formulated.

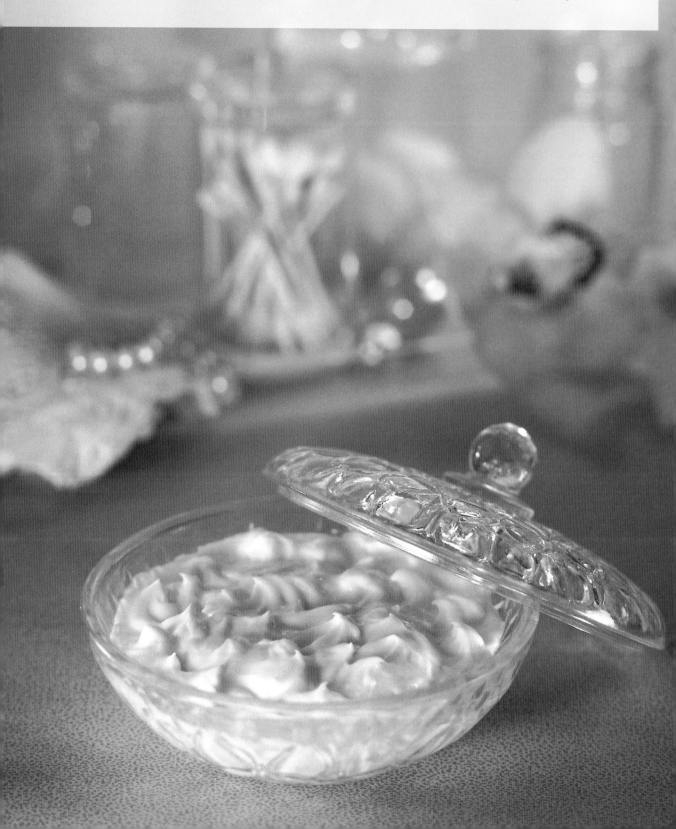

Tip: *Jojoba oil contains approximately four times the amount of waxy esters contained within the skin's sebum. Incorporating jojoba oil into skin creams not only protects the skin but allows the skin a chance to heal and repair itself.*

Creams

Face creams fall into two main types: moisturizers and cleansers. Although there are commercially available face cleansers that are clear, noncreamy liquids, these are often alcohol based. They effectively clean the face, but leave the skin dry and stripped of naturally occurring sebum. These are marketed at those with oily skin, or with acne, as they are supposed to reduce oiliness, but they only provide a temporary solution and are too harsh for the skin. Cream-based cleansers are much kinder to

the skin and they are equally effective at cleansing deep into the pores.

All moisturizing products are cream based. The process involves warming the fat-based ingredients—such as cocoa butter and almond oil—and the water-based ingredients— such as rose water or orange flower water—separately. These are then mixed together by dripping the latter slowly into the former, beating the mixture continuously.

Cocoa Butter and Rose Cream

This is a rich face cream that is especially suited to dry and mature skin. At the end of winter, when the face has been exposed to the drying effects of cold wind, rain, and central heating, the skin may be very dry and perhaps a little red or flaky. This lovely recipe contains both essential and base oils that have a gentle, deep, and lasting action on the skin, making the cream a really effective moisturizer.

what's in it?

1 tsp (4 gm) yellow beeswax	2 tbsp (35 ml) almond oil
½ cup (130 ml) rose water	1 tbsp (10 ml) jojoba oil
1 tbsp (10 ml) glycerin	15 drops rose
1½ tbsp (20 gm) cocoa butter	15 drops frankincense
	5 drops chamomile

how's it made?

1 Melt the beeswax in a bowl placed in a baking tray of hot water over a gentle heat.

2 Heat the rose water and glycerin in another bowl alongside the melting beeswax.

3 Once the beeswax has melted, add the cocoa butter, stirring constantly until it is melted. Then add the almond and jojoba oils, beating the mixture steadily to ensure all ingredients are thoroughly incorporated.

4 Once the contents of both bowls are the same temperature (warmed through but not simmering) add the

rose water and glycerin, drop by drop, into the oils. Beat steadily. An assistant can be useful at this stage, or you can even use an electric beater if you have one with a very low setting.

5 When all the rose water and glycerin have been beaten into the oils, remove from the heat, stirring until the mixture has cooled. Then add the essential oils, mixing them in thoroughly, and then pour into glass jars. Put the lids on once the cream is quite cool, label the jars, and the cream is ready to use.

Neroli and Petitgrain Cream Cleanser

This cleanser incorporates the nourishing oils of avocado and wheatgerm. Avocado oil regenerates skin cells and has skin softening and healing qualities. It is rich in vitamins A, D, and E, which are all beneficial for healthy skin. Wheatgerm oil contains carotene and vegetable lecithin, which help prevent moisture loss from the skin. The fragrance is delicate and floral.

what's in it?

½ oz (18 gm) yellow beeswax

4 tbsp (60 ml) orange flower water

4 tbsp (60 ml) avocado oil

2 tbsp (30 ml) wheatgerm oil

5 drops neroli

6 drops petitgrain

how's it made?

1 Melt the beeswax in a bowl placed in a baking tray of hot water over a gentle heat.

2 Heat the orange flower water in another small bowl alongside the melting beeswax.

3 Once the beeswax has melted, add the avocado and wheatgerm oils, beating the mixture to ensure the ingredients are thoroughly blended.

4 Once the contents of both bowls are the same temperature (warmed through but not simmering) add the orange flower water, drop by drop, into the oils. Beat steadily. An assistant can be useful at this stage, or you can even use an electric beater if you have one with a very low setting.

5 When all the flower water has been beaten into the oils, remove from the heat, stirring until the mixture has cooled. Then add the essential oils, mixing them in thoroughly, and then pour into glass jars. Put the lids on once the cream is quite cool, label the jars, and the cream is ready to use.

Almond Oil and Rosehip Seed Cream

The oil extracted from the Rosa Mosquetta rosehip seed is much valued for its skin-regeneration properties. Here, it is combined with almond oil to make a nourishing face cream suitable for all skin types. Delicate neroli is blended with lavender and a hint of ylang ylang to create a finely perfumed cream.

what's in it?

1½ tsp (5 gm) yellow beeswax	2 vitamin E capsules
1 tbsp (15 gm) rose water	10 drops neroli
2 tbsp (30 gm) almond oil	10 drops lavender
2 tsp (10 gm) rosehip seed oil, preferably Rosa Mosquetta	5 drops ylang ylang

how's it made?

1 Melt the beeswax in a bowl placed in a baking tray of hot water over a gentle heat.

2 Heat the rose water in another bowl alongside the melting beeswax.

3 Once the beeswax has melted, add the almond and rosehip seed oils, beating the mixture steadily to ensure they are incorporated thoroughly. Prick open the vitamin E capsules with a pin and squeeze into the mixture.

4 Once the contents of both bowls are the same temperature (warmed through but simmering) add the rose water, drop by drop, into the oils. Beat steadily. An assistant can be useful at this stage, or you can even use an electric beater if you have one with a very low setting.

5 When all the flower water has been beaten into the oils, remove from the heat, stirring until the mixture has cooled. Then add the essential oils, mixing them in thoroughly, and then pour into glass jars. Put the lids on once the cream is quite cool, label the jars, and the cream is ready to use.

Did You Know? *Wheatgerm oil is a natural antioxidant and it helps preserve the shelf life of the cream.*

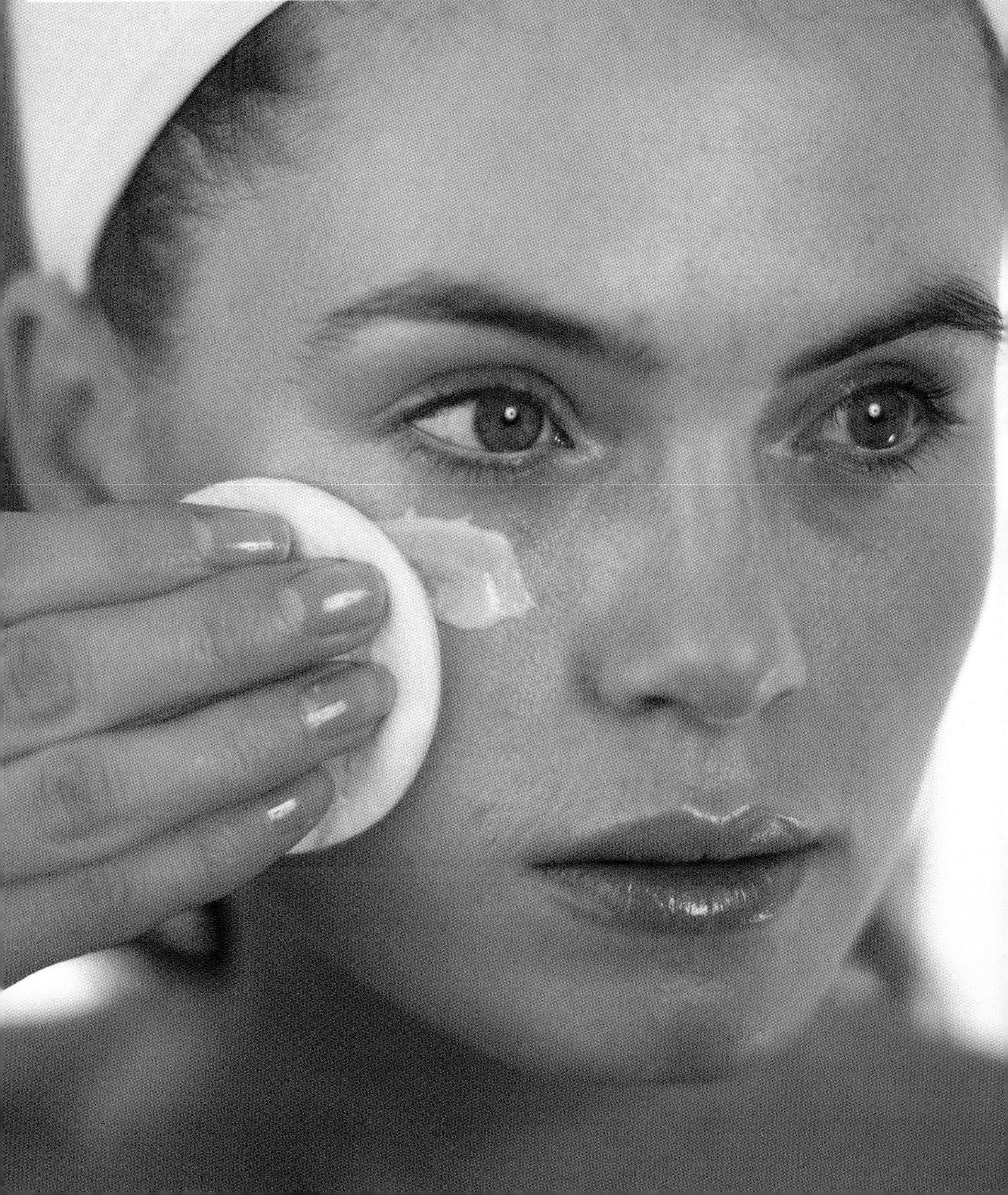

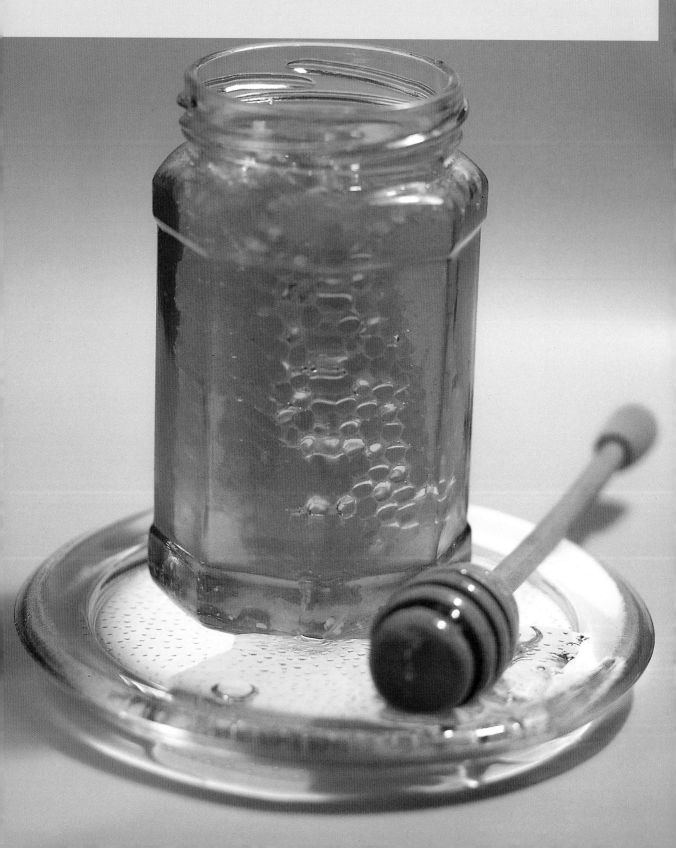

Shea Butter and Honey Antiwrinkle Cream

The healing properties of shea butter, or karite butter, have been used in skin care for centuries in central Africa. Shea butter has a gentle but effective moisturizing action, and is suitable for sensitive and dry skin that is prone to wrinkles. Combined with the healing properties of honey, this cream is a valuable cosmetic you will come to rely on to soften and soothe your skin.

what's in it?

2 tsp (7 gm) yellow beeswax	3 tsp (15 ml) almond oil
3 tsp (15 ml) linden flower water	2 tsp (10 ml) wheatgerm oil
1 tsp (5 ml) warmed liquid honey	2 drops myrrh
3 tsp (15 gm) shea butter	3 drops jasmine

how's it made?

1 Melt the beeswax in a bowl placed in a baking tray of hot water over a gentle heat.

2 Heat the linden flower water and honey in another bowl alongside the melting beeswax.

3 Once the beeswax has melted, add the shea butter, stirring constantly until it is melted. Then add the almond and wheatgerm oils, beating the mixture steadily to ensure all ingredients are thoroughly incorporated.

4 Once the contents of both bowls are the same temperature (warmed through but not simmering) add the linden flower water and honey, drop by drop, into the oils. Beat steadily. An assistant can be useful at this stage, or you can even use an electric beater if you have one with a very low setting.

5 When all the linden flower water and honey have been beaten into the oils, remove from the heat, stirring until the mixture has cooled. Then add the essential oils, mixing them in thoroughly, and then pour into glass jars. Put the lids on once the cream is quite cool, label the jars, and the cream is ready to use.

Galen's Cold Cream

This recipe is based on the original Galen's Cold Cream, which is thousands of years old. The cream sets firm but liquefies on contact with the natural warmth of the skin. Galen's Cold Cream is a good cleansing cream for mature and dry skin. Rose oil gives a wonderful and luxurious fragrance, making this cleanser a real treat to use.

what's in it?

2 tsp (10 gm) yellow beeswax

2 tbsp (30 gm) rose water

3 tbsp (40 gm) almond oil

10 drops rose

how's it made?

1 Melt the beeswax in a bowl placed in a baking tray of hot water over a gentle heat.

2 Heat the rose water in a second small bowl alongside the bowl of melting beeswax.

3 Once the beeswax has melted, add the almond oil, beating the mixture steadily to ensure the ingredients are thoroughly incorporated.

4 Once the contents of both bowls are the same temperature (warmed through but not simmering) add the rose water, drop by drop, into the oil. Beat steadily. An assistant can be useful at this stage, or you can use an electric beater if you have one with a very low setting.

5 When all the rose water has been beaten into the oil, remove from the heat, stirring until the mixture has cooled. Then add the rose, mixing it in thoroughly, and then pour into glass jars. Put the lids on once the cream is quite cool, label the jars, and the cream is ready to use.

Coconut Oil Hand Cream

This is a very simple cream to make as there is no flower water or beeswax to incorporate. The cream sets easily because coconut oil is solid at room temperature, but the cream easily liquefies on contact with the warmth of the skin. Lemon oil is fresh smelling and gently helps fade any discolored skin on the hands. It blends into a refreshing floral fragrance with the lavender.

what's in it?

5 tbsp (75 gm) coconut oil

1½ tbsp (25 gm) almond oil

10 drops lemon

10 drops lavender

how's it made?

1 Use a double boiler if you have one, or put a small saucepan inside a larger saucepan that is half filled with hot water. Add the coconut oil to the small saucepan and warm gently over a low heat until the coconut oil has melted.

2 Slowly pour in the almond oil, mixing continuously until the mixture is blended.

3 Remove from the heat and stir in the essential oils, mixing them in thoroughly, and pour into glass jars.

4 Put the lids on once the cream is quite cool, label the jars, and the cream is ready to use.

Geranium and Myrrh Hand Cream

This is another easy cream to make. It is excellent for those who work outdoors with their hands. The skin on the hands can easily become hard, dry, and chapped or cracked if it is not cared for properly. This hand cream is deeply penetrating and moisturizing, and the myrrh helps heal any small cuts, cracks, or lesions on the skin.

what's in it?

2 tsp (10 gm) yellow beeswax

4 tbsp (50 gm) cocoa butter

3 tbsp (40 ml) almond oil

1 tsp (5 ml) infused calendula oil

1 tsp (5 ml) glycerin

10 drops myrrh

10 drops geranium

how's it made?

1 Melt the beeswax in a bowl placed in a baking tray of hot water over a gentle heat.

2 Once the beeswax has melted, add the cocoa butter, stirring constantly until it is melted. Then add the almond oil and calendula oil, beating the mixture steadily to ensure all ingredients are thoroughly incorporated.

3 Add the glycerin to the oils in a slow trickle, beating steadily.

4 Once all the glycerin has been beaten into the oils, remove from the heat, stirring until the mixture has cooled. Then add the essential oils, mixing them in thoroughly, and then pour into glass jars. Put the lids on once the cream is quite cool, label the jars, and the cream is ready to use.

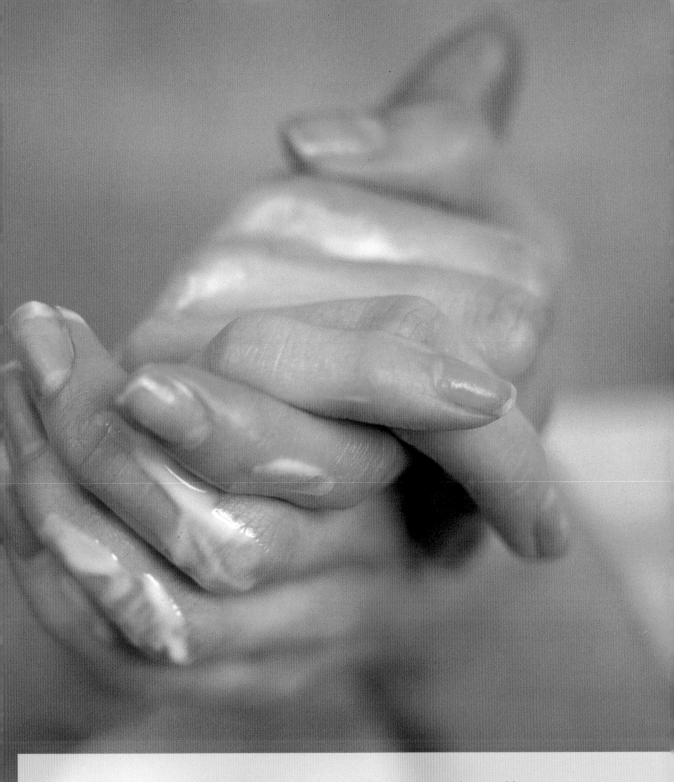

Tip: *Coconut Oil Hand Cream is also very good for the feet. After scrubbing away the hard, dead skin on the soles of the feet, apply the coconut oil cream for a deeply moisturizing treatment.*

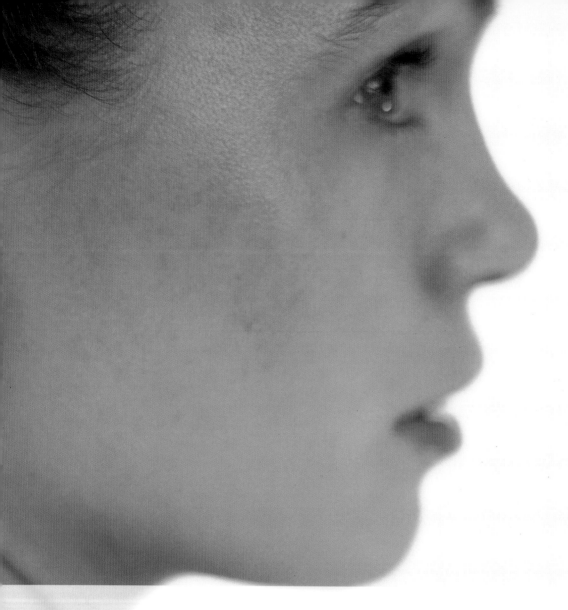

Tip: *Make sure you don't expose your skin to the sun immediately after using the lotion on page 49. It contains bergamot, a photosensitizer that could cause skin discoloration if used on the skin in strong sunlight.*

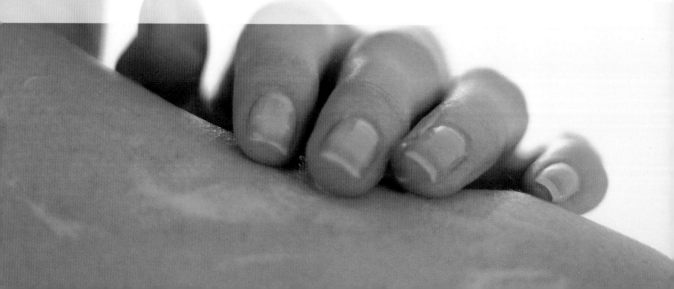

Lotions

Body lotions are moisturizers for the body. Lotions are thinner than face creams, so they spread easily over the larger areas of the body. Easy to apply, they are absorbed quickly by the skin. Body lotions are valuable in the summer when the sun has dried the skin, especially if you have been sunbathing. The body does need moisturizing all year round however, and body lotions provide a good way to moisturize the skin.

The following recipes can be made by using either a lotion base or thinning one of your homemade face or hand creams with flower water. Lotion base is ready to be used immediately in the recipes, and is quick and simple to use. If you would like to use one of your homemade creams, put a suitable quantity into a small glass jar. Put this in a container of hot water until the cream has softened or melted. Then beat in a flower water of your choice until you have the desired thickness of lotion. Use only half the quantity of nutrients and essential oils given in the recipe, as the cream already contains a proportion of these.

Light Body Lotion with Jasmine and Bergamot

This lotion is ideal to use in the winter months as an all over body lotion. The fragrance is floral and uplifting, and the light lotion is easily and quickly absorbed by the skin. Either use a light lotion base or thin down some Almond Oil and Rosehip Seed Cream (page 42) with orange flower water. Don't forget to halve the quantities in this recipe if you use thinned down face cream. Oat plant milk is a gentle, natural moisturizer that is easily absorbed by the skin.

what's in it?
6½ tbsp (100 ml) light lotion base

1 tsp (5 ml) cornflower water

4 tbsp (50 ml) oat plant milk

15 drops jasmine

5 drops petitgrain

10 drops bergamot

how's it made?

1 Pour the lotion base into a 8 or 10 oz (200 or 250 ml) glass bottle.

2 Pour the cornflower water into the bottle, put on the cap, and shake vigorously to thoroughly mix the ingredients. Then pour in the oat plant milk and shake well.

3 Carefully add the essential oils into the bottle, one by one, then put on the cap and shake vigorously.

4 Label the bottle and the Light Body Lotion with Jasmine and Bergamot is ready to use.

After Sun Body Lotion

This lotion is also good for dry and sensitive skin in addition to use after sunbathing. After the skin has been exposed to the sun, it tends to soak up lotions very quickly. It's important to use this lotion sparingly to prevent overloading your body with too much essential oil. If your skin needs more lotion after one application, use plain body lotion base, and return to using the After Sun lotion the following day.

what's in it?

¾ cup (150 ml) rich lotion base	5 drops neroli
	5 drops lavender
1 tsp (5 ml) rose water	5 drops sandalwood
1 tsp (5 ml) infused carrot seed oil	5 drops frankincense
10 drops chamomile	

how's it made?

1 Pour the lotion base into a 8 or 10 oz (200 or 250 ml) glass bottle.

2 Pour the rose water into the bottle, put on the cap, and shake vigorously to thoroughly mix the ingredients. Then add the carrot oil and shake well.

3 Carefully add the essential oils into the bottle, one by one, then put on the cap and shake vigorously.

4 Label the bottle and the After Sun Body Lotion is now ready to use.

Rich Body Lotion with Avocado Oil

Powerful and revitalizing essential oils combine with a rich lotion base and avocado oil to make an effective and luxurious body lotion. The fragrance is sumptuous and exotic, and this is a wonderful lotion to use after an evening bath for a romantic evening. This lotion is suitable for all skin types and works especially well on mature and dry skin.

what's in it?

¾ cup (150 ml) rich lotion base	10 drops patchouli
	5 drops neroli
1 teaspoon Monoi de Tahiti	5 drops rose
1 tsp (5 ml) rose water	5 drops vanilla
1 tsp (5 ml) avocado oil	5 drops orange

how's it made?

1 Pour the lotion base into a 8 or 10 oz (200 or 250 ml) glass bottle. Warm the bottle in a mug of hot water. Melt the Monoi de Tahiti in a small dish in the microwave and add to the bottle. Shake well.

2 Pour the rose water into the bottle, put on the cap, and shake vigorously to thoroughly mix the ingredients. Then add the avocado oil and shake well.

3 Carefully add the essential oils into the bottle, one by one, then put on the cap and shake vigorously.

4 Label the bottle and the Rich Body Lotion with Avocado Oil is now ready to use.

Did You Know? *Avocado oil is rich and nourishing and works especially well on mature and dry skin, helping to prevent wrinkles.*

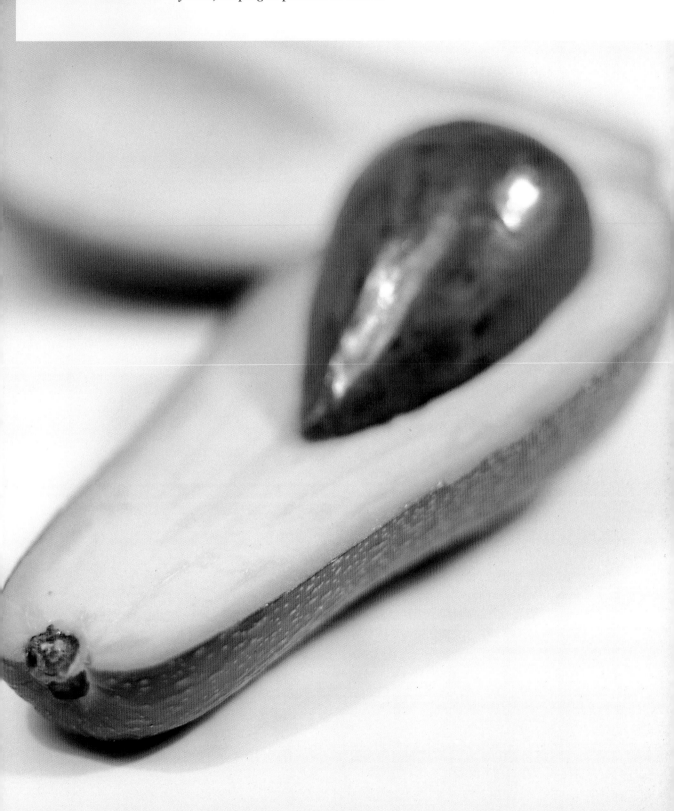

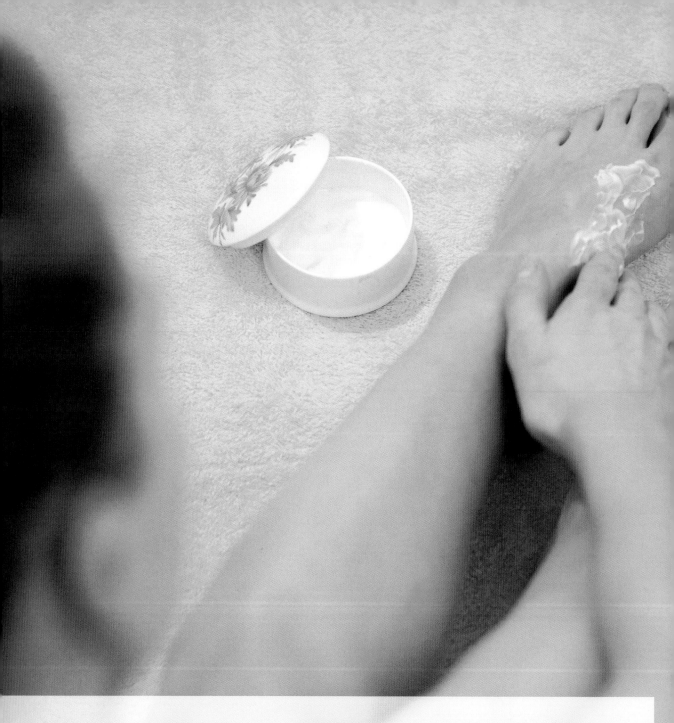

Tip: *This home pedicure keeps your feet looking good as well as feeling good. Do it once a week for a month before going on your summer vacation and your feet will look great.*

Peppermint Foot Lotion

Our feet do a hard job for us every day, carrying our body weight and frequently walking long distances. This stimulating and refreshing foot lotion is a great way to revive and rejuvenate tired feet. Soak your feet in a bowl of hot water for ten minutes, then scrub off any dead skin. Gently rub your feet with this lotion and they will feel wonderful afterwards!

what's in it?

¾ cup (150 ml) light lotion base

1 tsp (5 ml) orange flower water

15 drops peppermint

5 drops lemon

5 drops cypress

5 drops juniper

how's it made?

1 Pour the lotion base into a 8 or 10 oz (200 or 250 ml) glass bottle.

2 Pour the orange flower water into the bottle, put on the cap, and shake vigorously to thoroughly mix the ingredients.

3 Carefully add the essential oils into the bottle, one by one, then put on the cap and shake vigorously.

4 Label the bottle and the Peppermint Foot Lotion is now ready to use.

Lip Balms

Lip balms are indispensable in the winter to avoid sore, chapped lips. Although lipsticks can protect your lips to some extent, many people prefer lip balms, as they are usually made without the use of animal fats. It also means you can protect your lips without coloring them as well.

Homemade lip balms are really effective. Using a natural, organic base and infused oils, essential oils, and beeswax, you can create nourishing lip balms that will protect your lips against the drying effects of cold, wind, and central heating.

The following recipes make enough to fill five small, ½ oz (15 gm) glass jars. You could also use ornamental ceramic pots, if you prefer. Avoid using one large jar as the lip balm will keep better in smaller containers.

Aniseed and Lemon Lip Balm

This is a tangy, refreshing lip balm that leaves a fresh, clean taste on your lips. The base of almond and apricot oils gently lubricates and moisturizes the lips, while the vitamin E is good for regenerating the lips' delicate skin.

what's in it?

5 drops yellow color base (see step 1)

2 tbsp (30 ml) calendula oil

4 tbsp (50 ml) sweet almond oil

2 tbsp (25 ml) apricot kernel oil

1 drop liquid honey

1 tbsp (12 gm) beeswax pellets

2 vitamin E capsules

2 drops aniseed

3 drops lemon

how's it made?

1 Make the yellow color base by adding one teaspoon of ground turmeric to one tablespoon of sunflower oil in a small cup. Heat over boiling water or in a microwave until it bubbles, then remove from heat and pour into a dropper bottle.

2 Prepare a double boiler (one saucepan that fits inside another) by filling the bottom half with hot water and heating to a gentle simmer.

3 Measure out the base oils, one by one, and pour into the top half of the boiler.

4 Add the honey, beeswax pellets, and yellow color base. Stir gently to mix the ingredients.

5 As the beeswax is melting, prick open the vitamin E capsules and squeeze the contents into the oils.

6 Once the beeswax has fully melted remove from the heat. Drop in the aniseed and lemon and stir to mix them in thoroughly.

7 Pour into small glass jars or ceramic pots, and let cool for half an hour or until set. The lip balm is ready to use.

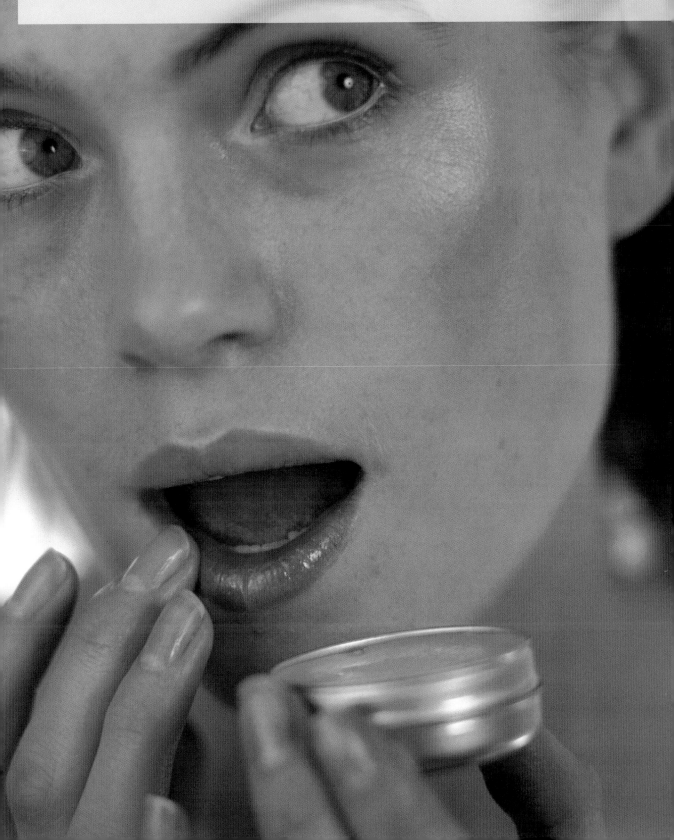

Tip: *The yellow color base gives the impression of lemon, but you could use a brown color base if you prefer, as this gives the impression of aniseed. Alternatively, you can omit the color altogether.*

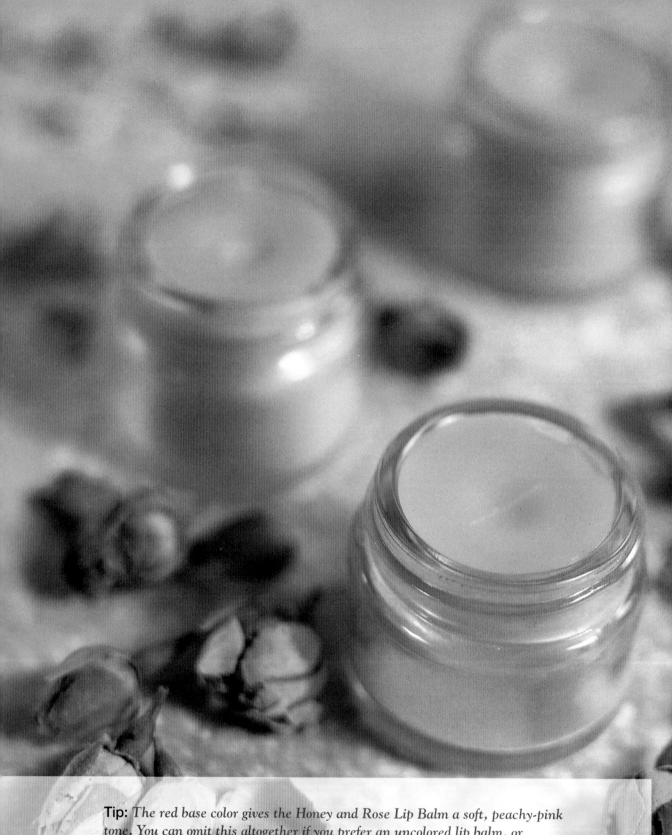

Tip: *The red base color gives the Honey and Rose Lip Balm a soft, peachy-pink tone. You can omit this altogether if you prefer an uncolored lip balm, or increase the number of drops to achieve a deeper shade of color.*

Honey and Rose Lip Balm

The delicate smell of roses combines with the sweetness of honey to make a truly scrumptious and luxurious lip balm. The use of healing calendula oil soothes and heals chapped lips, while the rosehip oil keeps the lips smooth and moisturized.

what's in it?

5 drops red color base (see step 1)	1 drop liquid honey
1 tbsp (15 ml) rosehip seed oil	1 tbsp (12 gm) beeswax pellets
1 tbsp (15 ml) calendula oil	2 vitamin E capsules
5 tbsp (75 ml) sweet almond oil	5 drops rose

how's it made?

1 Make the red color base by adding one teaspoon of ground alkanet root to one tablespoon of sunflower oil in a small cup. Heat over boiling water or in a microwave until it bubbles, then remove from heat and pour into a dropper bottle.

2 Prepare the double boiler (one saucepan that fits inside another) by filling the bottom half with hot water and heating to a gentle simmer.

3 Measure out the base oils, one by one, and pour into the top half of the boiler.

4 Add the honey, beeswax pellets, and red color base. Stir gently to mix the ingredients.

5 As the beeswax is melting, prick open the vitamin E capsules and squeeze the contents into the oils.

6 Once the beeswax has fully melted, remove from the heat. Drop in the rose and stir to mix it in thoroughly.

7 Pour into small glass jars or ceramic pots, and let cool for half an hour or until set. The lip balm is ready to use.

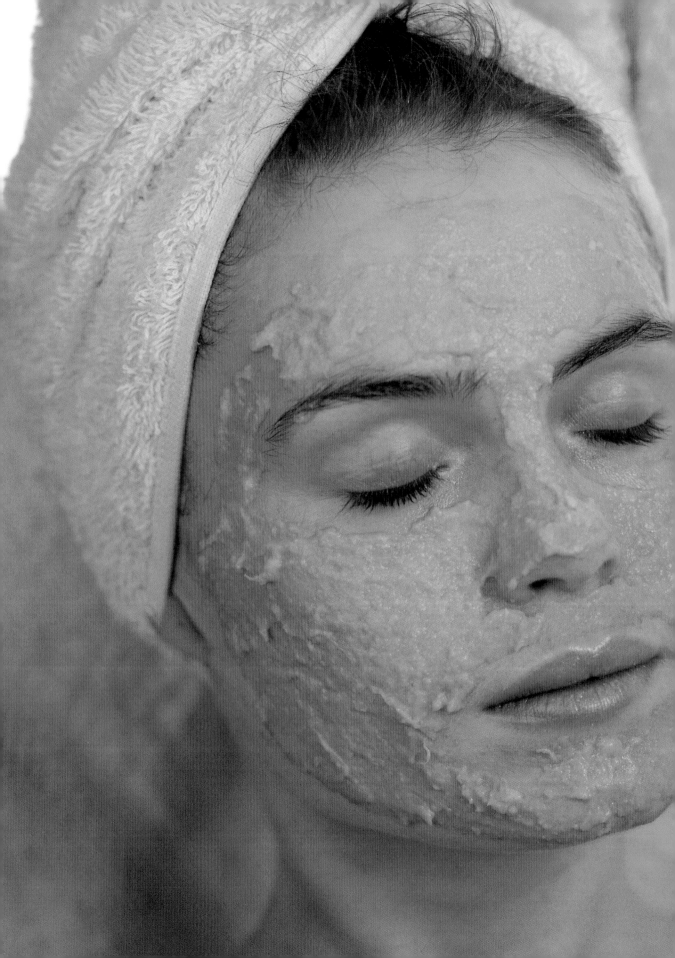

Chapter 4

Face Masks and Rejuvenating Treatments

"Dull skin, rough hands, and so forth will not inspire confidence."
–Patricia Davis, *author and aromatherapist*

Organic Beauty Treatments

Skin creams and lotions moisturize the skin and can be used daily as part of a skin-care regime alongside cleansers and toners. However, we need specialized rejuvenating treatments once a week or month to keep our face and body looking and feeling in tip-top condition. In this chapter, you will find recipes for face masks, exfoliating scrubs, and a luxurious and rejuvenating bath milk.

Face masks are a major rejuvenating treatment. They are applied to the face and the neck—take care to avoid the eyes, the surrounding delicate skin, and the mouth—and left for ten or fifteen minutes to do their work. Masks serve one of several purposes, depending on the ingredients used. Some masks are enriching and nourishing, feeding and hydrating the skin. Ingredients for these masks include honey, almond, and avocado.

Sadly, face masks alone won't transform your skin into the dewy complexion of a model! So, it is a good idea to spend a day detoxifying from the inside as well as from the outside. If you choose a day when you don't have to work, you can really rest and revitalize your whole system. During the day, avoid all caffeine, salt, chemical additives, and alcohol. Drink herb teas and a lot of spring water. Eat a lot of fruit—melons and grapes are especially good for detoxifying your system. Make a simple vegetable soup for lunch and in the evening steam some organic vegetables and serve them with organic brown rice.

As well as applying one of the face masks that follow, you can thoroughly cleanse and tone your face beforehand and give yourself a face massage. In one teaspoon of almond oil put a single drop of rose, jasmine, or neroli. Massage this gently into your face and neck, avoiding the eyes and mouth. After the massage, rest for five minutes with a warm, damp cloth over your face. Then, apply your chosen face mask and rest for ten or fifteen minutes before washing it off with warm water.

Skin benefits from regular exfoliation, and a recipe for a body scrub is also provided. This is important in the spring, as your body has been swathed in thick clothes and subject to the drying effects of wind and central heating. However, regular exfoliation year round keeps the skin in good condition, vibrantly glowing, and healthy.

The feet benefit from a coarser scrub than the rest of the body as the skin is thicker. Use a handful of sea salt, and rub firmly in circular movements, targeting the areas of hard skin. Wash off the salt with warm water and then apply the Peppermint Foot Lotion or Coconut Oil Hand Cream (see pages 53 and 46, respectively), or give yourself a foot massage with a few drops of an essential oil of your choice mixed into a teaspoon of almond oil.

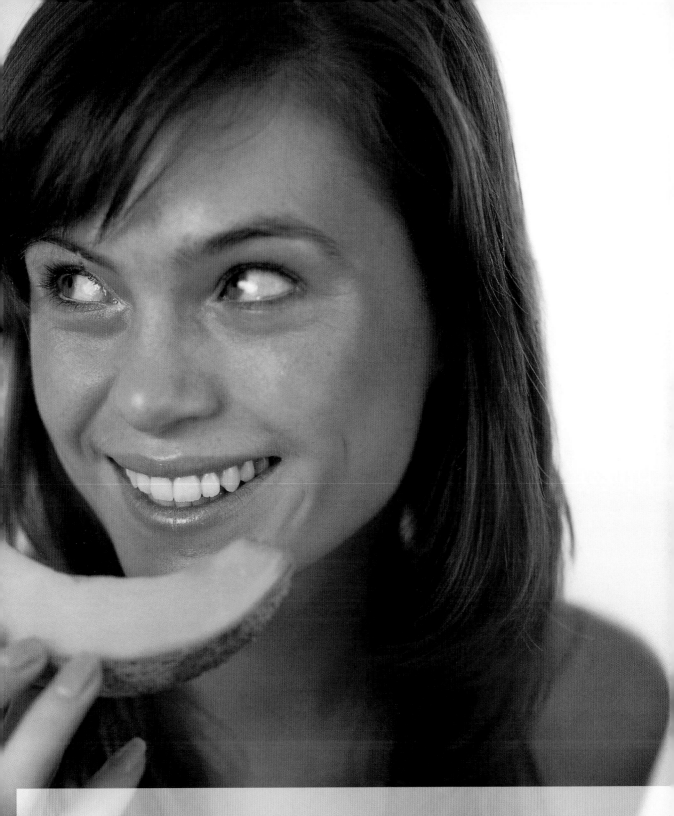

Tip: *While face masks will help nourish your skin, you should also take time to detoxify from the inside as well. To this end, make sure you eat lots of organic fresh fruit, especially melons.*

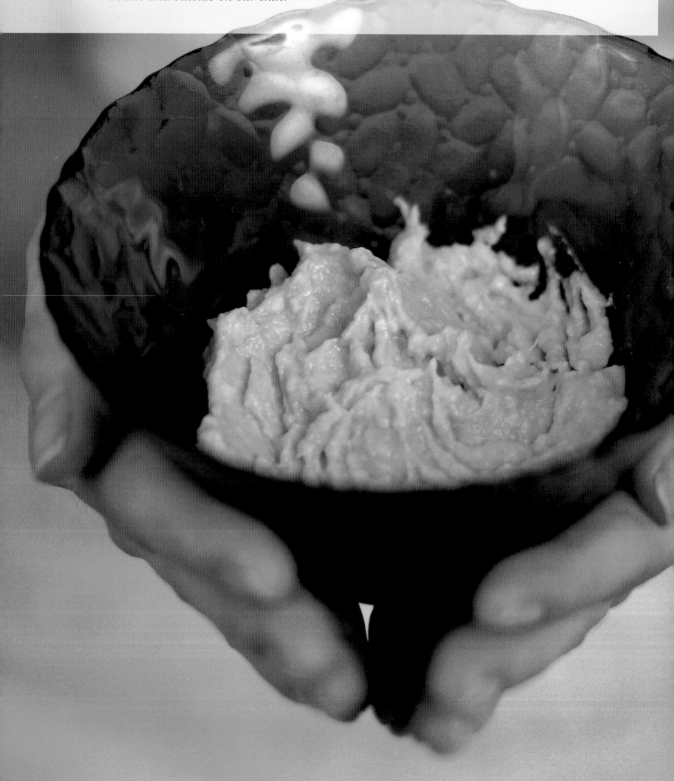

Tip: *If there is any avocado leftover from making the face mask, don't waste it—eat it! Avocado is one of nature's gifts and is good for our health, both inside our bodies and outside on our skin.*

Face Masks

Following are recipes for face masks, including a deep cleansing mask with green clay and a skin nourishing mask with almonds and honey. Check the condition of your skin, as well as your skin type, before choosing which face mask to use. Does your skin look dull and need a deep cleanse? Or perhaps your skin feels tired and dry and needs a nourishing mask?

Homemade face masks are fun but messy, so make sure you have plenty of old towels around. Also, before you start, decide where you will rest once the mask is applied. Lying down is best, as it stops the mask from slipping off your face. You can make eye pads to cover your eyes. Either soak cotton pads in rose water or keep a couple of cooled, used chamomile tea bags and use these instead.

Avocado Enriching Face Mask

This is one of the simplest face masks to make as it only has one ingredient! Avocado is very nourishing for the skin, and this mask is especially good for mature, wrinkled, and dry skin, although it is suitable for all skin types. Make sure you use a ripe, fresh, organic avocado for the best effect.

what's in it?
1 very ripe, organic avocado

how's it made?

1 Peel the avocado and remove the stone. Chop up the avocado and put it in a small glass bowl.

2 Using a fork, mash the avocado to a creamy pulp, making sure you break down any lumps.

3 Apply the avocado mask immediately to a cleansed face, and rest for ten minutes.

4 Finally, wash off the mask with warm water and apply a toner and moisturizer.

Honey and Almond Moisturizing Face Mask

The combination of honey and ground almonds makes this mask smell good enough to eat! Although it feels very sticky, and takes a lot of washing off, this is nonetheless a wonderful face mask, and worth the effort. The honey and almond moisturizing face mask is particularly good for mature, sensitive, or dry skin, but is suitable for all skin types.

what's in it?

1 large tsp honey
1 tbsp ground almonds
Enough warm water to mix to a spreadable paste

how's it made?

1 Warm the honey in a small bowl immersed in hot water until it becomes liquid.

2 Put the ground almonds into another small bowl. Add the melted honey and mix well, adding a little warm water to obtain a spreadable consistency.

3 Immediately apply the mask to a cleansed face and rest for ten to fifteen minutes.

4 Finally, wash off the mask with warm water and apply a toner and moisturizer.

Yogurt and Oatmeal Deep Cleansing Face Mask

Yogurt has been used for centuries for its health giving properties. Here, live, organic yogurt is mixed with finely ground oatmeal and a little honey for an all purpose face mask. This face mask is suited to all skin types, and is both cleansing and rejuvenating. If you have any doubt about which face mask to use, this is the one to go for.

what's in it?

1 tbsp finely ground oatmeal
1 tbsp live, organic yogurt
1 small tsp honey

how's it made?

1 Place the oatmeal in a bowl. Add the yogurt and mix to a spreadable consistency.

2 Warm the honey in a small glass bowl. Pour into the yogurt and oatmeal mixture and blend the ingredients thoroughly.

3 Immediately apply the yogurt and oatmeal mask to a cleansed face and rest for ten to fifteen minutes.

4 Finally, wash off the mask with warm water and apply a toner and moisturizer.

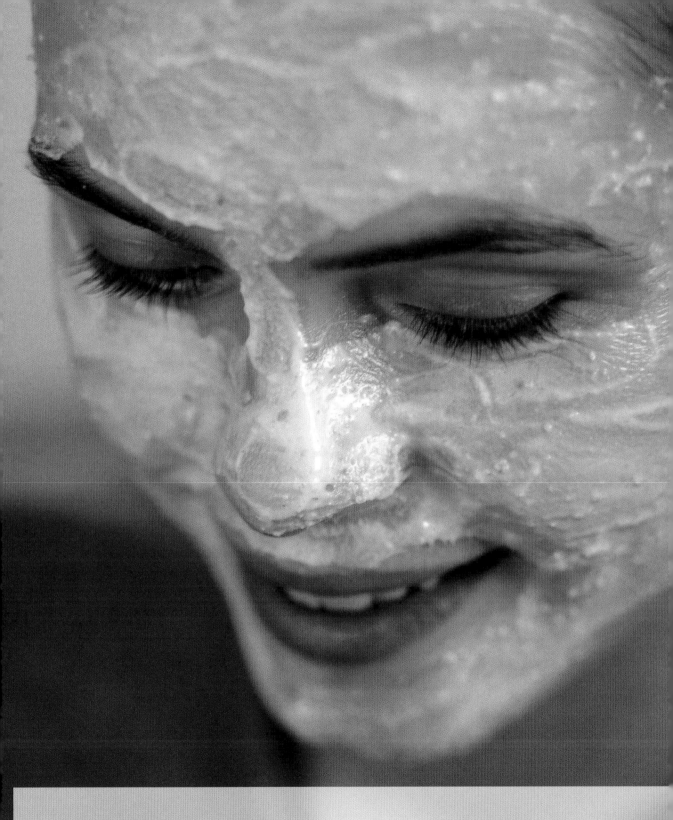

Did You Know? *Yogurt has a softening effect on the skin and a very mild bleaching action, helping to dispel skin blemishes.*

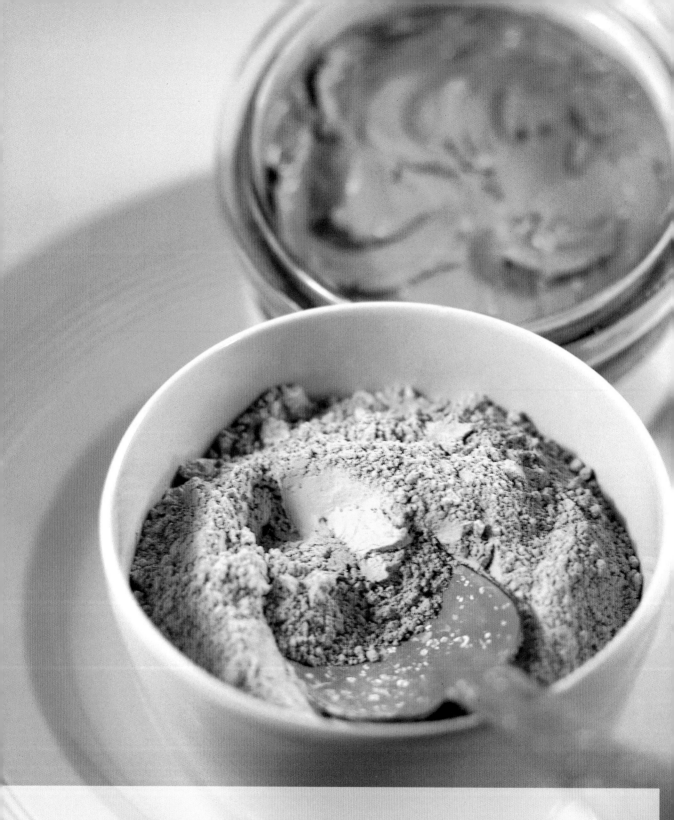

Tip: *If you have dry skin but would like to use the green clay mask, double the quantity of the apricot oil.*

Green Clay Purifying Mask

Green clay is also known as bentonite, and is the most commonly used clay in face masks. It has a slippery feel and can absorb large quantities of water. This mask is used to draw out excess sebum, toxins, and dirt from deep down in the skin and is best suited to oily skin. Green clay stabilizes the production of sebum and deeply cleanses the skin.

what's in it?

1 tsp apricot kernel oil

2 drops palmarosa

1 tbsp green clay

Enough warm water to mix to a spreadable paste

how's it made?

1 Mix the apricot oil and the palmarosa together in small dish.

2 Put the green clay in a small bowl. Add the apricot oil mixture and stir. Add just enough warm water to make a spreadable paste, and work the mixture thoroughly to incorporate all the ingredients.

3 Immediately apply the mask to a cleansed face and rest for ten to fifteen minutes. The mask will tighten slightly as the water evaporates and may feel a little strange. Don't worry; it's just the mask doing its work.

4 Finally, wash off the mask with warm water and apply a toner and moisturizer.

Rejuvenating Treatments

These rejuvenating treatments are designed to restore the skin's natural bloom. The body scrub achieves this effect by exfoliation, the removal of the skin's surface of dead skin cells, revealing the fresh new skin underneath. Exfoliation also stimulates the circulation, bringing more blood and nutrients to the skin and carrying away the toxins. Ideally, you should have a body scrub once a month, but even an occasional scrub will leave you with lovely skin for a while.

The bath milk and face oil are luxurious moisturizing treatments that deeply penetrate the skin with enriching, nourishing oils that help the skin retain its natural elasticity and restore its smooth, glowing appearance. The nutrients and oils combine to create rejuvenating treatments that leave you feeling invigorated and give you silky smooth skin that also smells divine. These two treatments are easier to make up and use than the body scrub, and you could aim to do them once a week.

Rejuvenating Rose Bath Milk

Bathing in milk is an ancient beauty treatment, first popularized by Cleopatra, who took weekly baths of assess' milk. These days, there are available store-bought bath milks already fragranced, and base bath milks that you can customize with essential oils. This recipe also contains the nourishing natural moisturizing properties of almonds and the rejuvenating effect of pure, organic rose oil.

what's in it?

2 tsp (10 gm) ground almonds
6½ tbsp (100 ml) rose water
6½ tbsp (100 ml) bath milk base
50 drops rose

how's it made?

1 Place the ground almonds and rose water in a blender. Blend for a couple of minutes. Let the mixture stand for a few minutes, then blend again for a couple of minutes. Repeat once more.

2 Strain the rose and almond milk through fine muslin into a container, then pour into a 9 oz (250 ml) glass bottle.

3 Add the bath milk base and shake well. Carefully count in the drops of rose, and shake well so all the ingredients are thoroughly blended.

4 Label the bottle and the Rejuvenating Rose Bath Milk is ready to use. For each bath, pour in one or two tablespoons of bath milk.

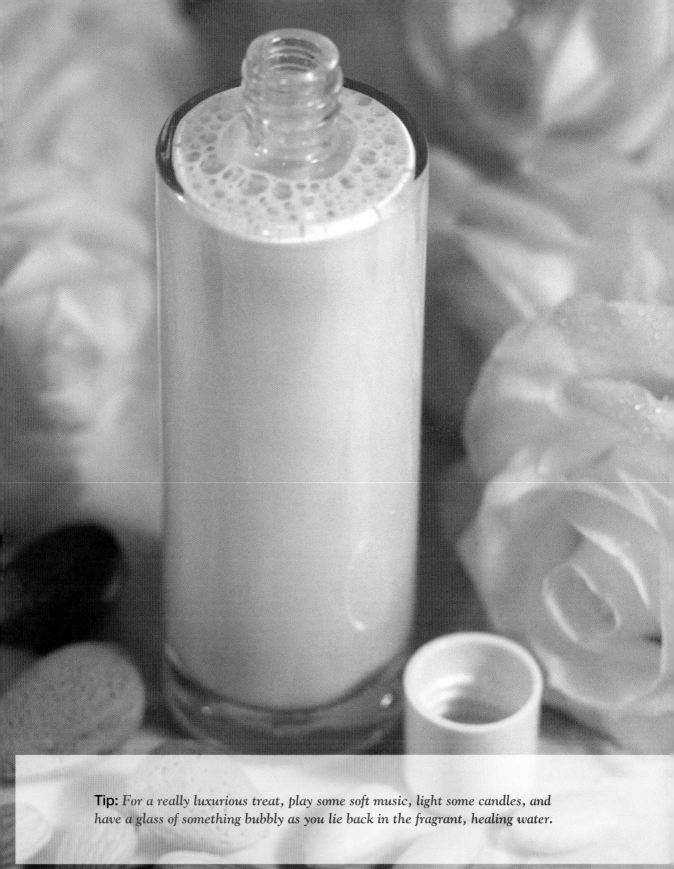

Tip: *For a really luxurious treat, play some soft music, light some candles, and have a glass of something bubbly as you lie back in the fragrant, healing water.*

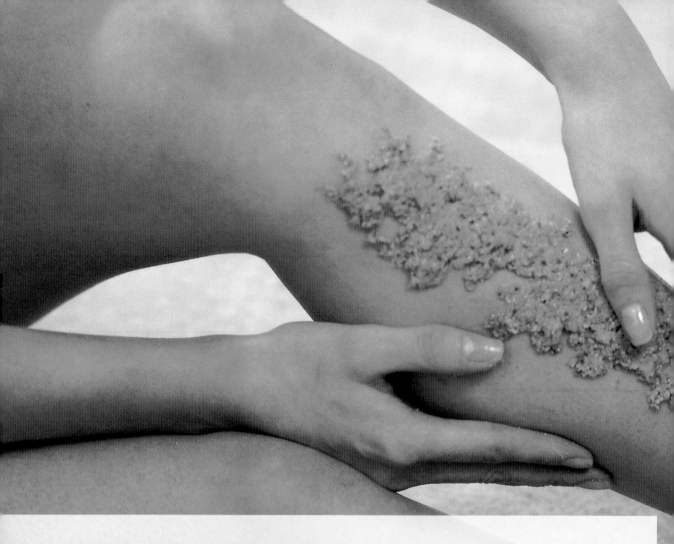

Tip: *You could try doing the Rejuvenating, Exfoliating Body Scrub with your partner or friend, as it is easier to scrub someone else than to scrub yourself, though it is fine to do by yourself too. It's best to do the body scrub standing in the bath, as it's a messy procedure.*

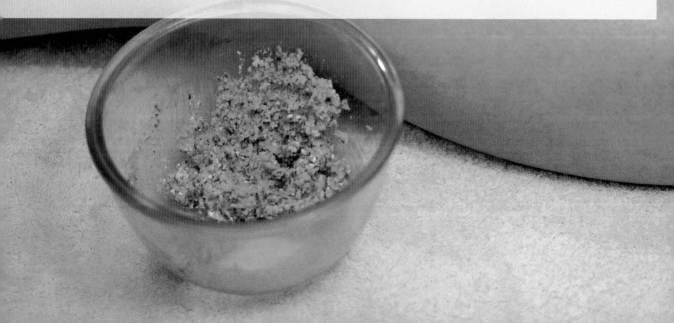

Rejuvenating, Exfoliating Body Scrub

This rejuvenating treatment is based on a traditional Indian body scrub for brides. The bride is scrubbed all over with a traditional mixture of finely ground grains, fruit peels, spices, and oils, and then she is massaged with sweet smelling oils. This is performed daily for ten days, so at the wedding she looks wonderful with smooth, sweet smelling skin. Using this body scrub will leave you with glowing skin.

what's in it?

2 tbsp fine ground oatmeal

2 tbsp ground almonds

1 tsp dried, finely ground orange peel

1 tsp rosehip granules

5 drops jasmine

Enough warm water to moisten the mixture

how's it made?

1 Place all the dried ingredients in a large bowl and mix thoroughly.

2 Add the jasmine and a little warm water to make a fine, crumbly mixture. Don't use too much water or you will end up with a sticky mess.

3 Stand in the bathtub or on a towel spread over the floor. Take a small handful of the body scrub and scrub vigorously with circular movements all over the body. Be systematic; do the legs and arms first as they are easiest, and then do as much of the rest of your body as you can reach.

4 The scrub dries quickly, and most of it will fall off your body. When you have finished, use a soft body brush to brush off any leftover crumbs.

Rejuvenating Face Oil

Although this face oil takes a little longer than a face cream to be absorbed into the skin, using this rejuvenating face oil once a week will literally feed your face with exceptional nutrients. Make sure you have thoroughly cleansed and toned your face before applying the face oil. You don't need a moisturizing face cream, as the face oil itself is deeply moisturizing.

what's in it?

1 tbsp (10 ml) kukui nut oil	3 evening primrose oil
1 tbsp (10 ml) jojoba oil	capsules
1 tbsp (10 ml) apricot	4 drops rose
kernel oil	3 drops neroli
1 tsp (5 ml) almond oil	3 drops jasmine
1 tsp (5 ml) avocado oil	3 drops frankincense
1 tbsp (10 ml) rosehip oil	2 drops sandalwood

how's it made?

1 Carefully measure out and pour all the base oils into a 2 or 3 oz (75 or 100 ml) dark glass bottle. Shake well.

2 With a pin, prick open the capsules of evening primrose oil and squeeze in to the bottle.

3 Carefully add in the essential oils, one by one. Shake the bottle well.

4 Label the bottle. The Rejuvenating Face Oil is ready to use.

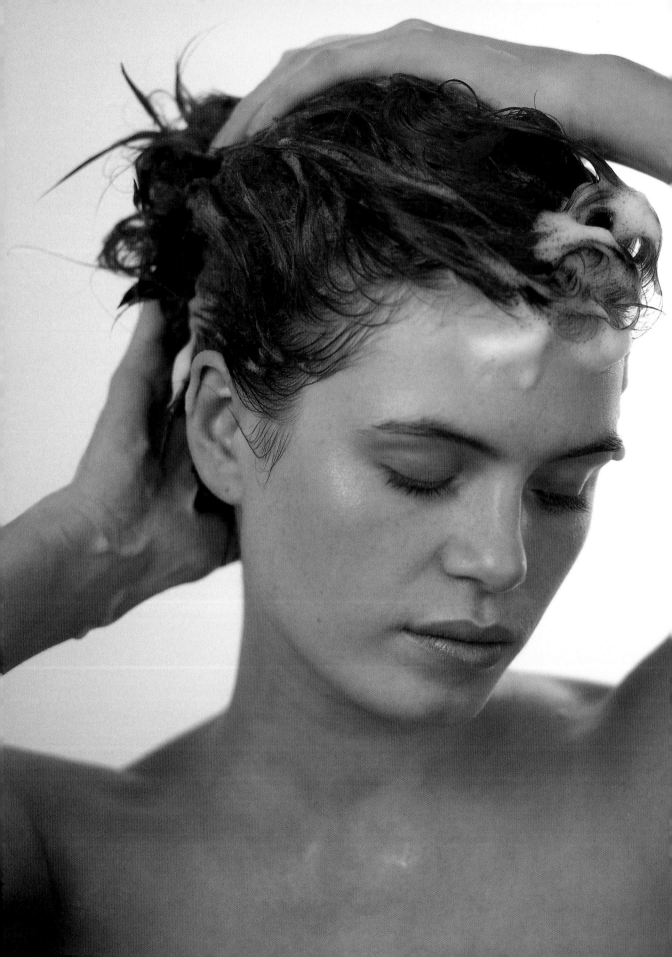

Chapter 5

Hair Shampoos and Conditioners

"Synthetics have intruded upon all areas of our lives—we need only read the back of our shampoo bottle for an example."
—Susan Miller Cavitch, *natural soap maker and author*

Homemade Hair Care

Our hair is mainly composed of a protein called keratin, which also forms our fingernails and the outer layer of our skin. Keratin is actually dead tissue, produced as the living cells—including those in the hair root, or follicle—die and are replaced by new cells. This means the health of your hair depends on the health of the hair follicles, from which the hair grows. The hair follicles depend on a good supply of oxygen from the surrounding blood vessels, so to keep your hair in good condition you need to stimulate circulation in the scalp by regular head massage.

You already do a little massage when you shampoo your hair, and using a hair brush is also stimulating for the scalp. However, if you would like to improve the condition of your hair, try doing a scalp massage daily for five minutes or so. Use small, firm, circular movements with your fingertips, and make sure you move the scalp itself, so you are not just massaging your hair.

No oil is required for this scalp massage, but doing a massage with oil once a week will condition the hair and scalp, although you will have to wash your hair afterward. Take one teaspoon of warmed almond oil and add three drops of essential oil. Dip your fingers frequently into this mixture as you do the scalp massage. If you have dark hair,

use rosemary; for fair hair, use chamomile; and if you suffer from dandruff, use sandalwood, lavender, or bergamot.

Our hair benefits from natural, organic, plant-based products as much as our face and body. Many store-bought shampoos are harsh, and although they leave the hair clean, they strip off the natural coating of sebum. Sebum is our own natural moisturizer; an oily wax produced by glands in the body and in the hair follicles.

Shampoo and conditioner bases can be bought from one of the suppliers listed on pages 222–223. These shampoos and conditioners are made from natural plant material—often organic—and contain no chemical additives. This means they are exceptionally mild, and leave the hair clean but not stripped completely of sebum.

The mildness of these plant-based hair-care products also means the scalp is cared for and not aggravated by harsh cleansers or chemicals. If you are prone to an itchy or flakey scalp, switching to your own homemade shampoos and conditioners could well relieve you of these unpleasant symptoms. After a few weeks of using these mild, natural hair treatments you are likely to have a healthy scalp and soft, glossy hair.

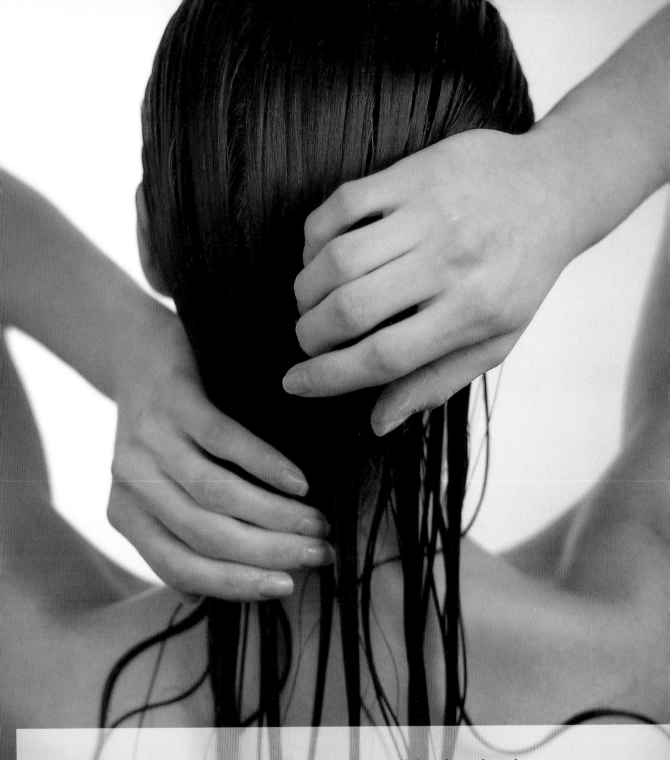

Did You Know? When we brush our hair, we spread the sebum along the individual hair shafts, and it is this that keeps our hair shiny, smooth, and glossy. Without the protective coating of sebum, the hair becomes dull, brittle, and lifeless, and the hair ends are prone to splitting.

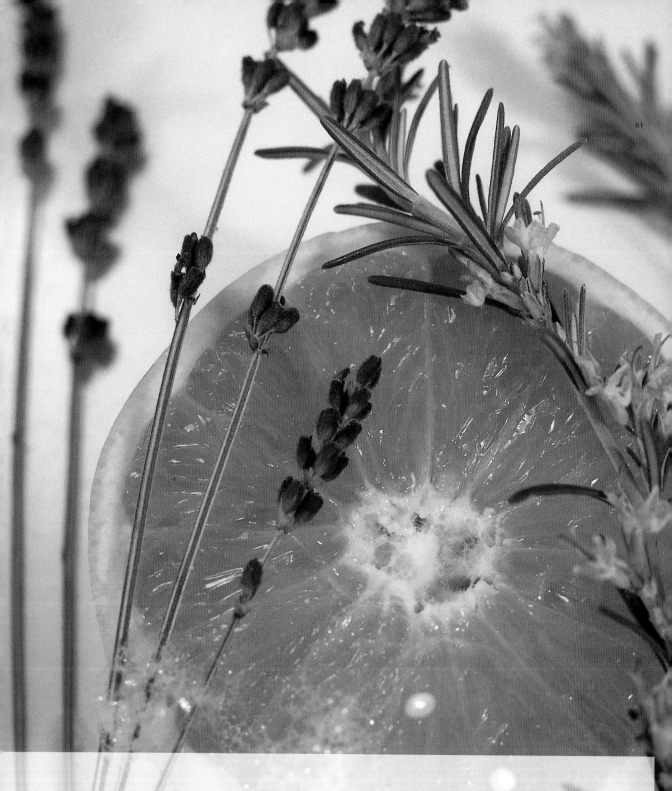

Did You Know? When citrus oils are blended into shampoo, they leave your hair smelling incredibly fresh and clean.

Shampoos

Caring for your hair and scalp is easy when you use mild shampoos enriched and perfumed with essential oils. Buying your shampoo base from a supplier of natural cosmetic products ensures you will get a high-quality, mild, natural, plant-based shampoo. Instead of harsh detergents and chemicals, the shampoo will be made from mild soaps, together with emulsifiers, nutrients, and so forth. These combine to make a shampoo gentle enough for even the most sensitive skin and hair damaged by bleaching or coloring.

Some suppliers offer organic base products, and by adding organic essential oils you will end up with a shampoo that will really care for and protect your hair and scalp in addition to cleaning them thoroughly. Your homemade shampoos are gentle enough to use on a daily basis, if required.

Herbal Shampoo with Pine and Grapefruit

This is a traditional herbal shampoo with the added zing of pine and grapefruit. Lavender and rosemary are often used in shampoos. Lavender calms and soothes the scalp, and rosemary and pine are stimulating, helping bring blood, which is rich in nutrients, to the scalp. Grapefruit has a tonic effect on the skin and scalp and the delightful smell makes a welcome addition to this shampoo. Herbal shampoo is particularly recommended for oily hair but is suitable for all hair types.

what's in it?
6½ tbsp (100 ml) shampoo base
10 drops lavender
10 drops rosemary
5 drops pine
5 drops grapefruit

how's it made?

1 Pour the shampoo base into a glass container with a good pouring spout.

2 Carefully add the essential oils, one by one. Use a glass stirring rod or a chopstick to thoroughly stir the oils.

3 Pour into a glass bottle, plastic squeeze bottle, or pump dispenser using a funnel to avoid spillage.

4 Label the bottle and the herbal shampoo is ready to use.

Chamomile and Geranium Shampoo

This delightful smelling shampoo is a good general shampoo for all hair types but is especially good for dry hair. The combination of chamomile, sandalwood, and geranium provides a restorative effect, helping balance the production of sebum. This shampoo helps restore vitality to dull and lifeless hair, giving a long lasting shine.

what's in it?

6½ tbsp (100 ml) shampoo base
10 drops chamomile
10 drops geranium
5 drops sandalwood
3 drops lemon
2 drops lime

how's it made?

1 Pour the shampoo base into a glass container with a good pouring spout.

2 Carefully add the essential oils, one by one. Use a glass stirring rod or a chopstick to thoroughly stir the oils.

3 Pour into a glass bottle, plastic squeeze bottle, or pump dispenser using a funnel to avoid spillage.

4 Label the bottle and the Chamomile and Geranium Shampoo is ready to use.

Tip: *All essential oils are antiseptic to some extent, but pine is especially effective. Its refreshing and deodorant properties are often used in bathing and cleansing products.*

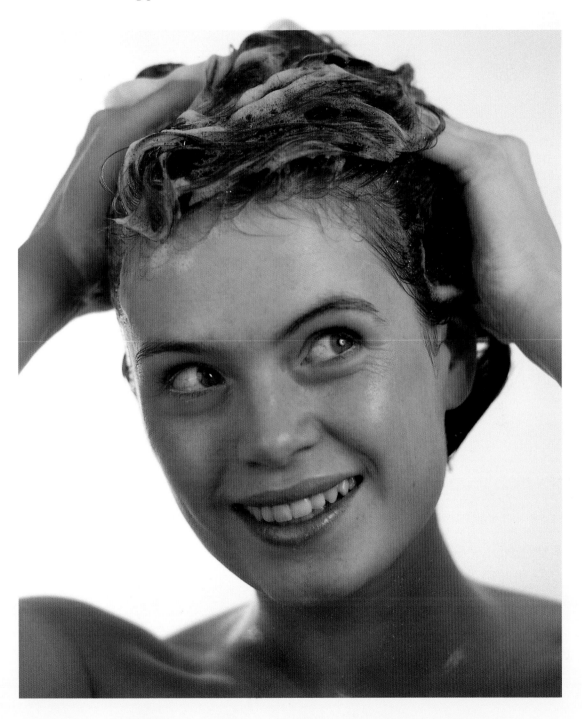

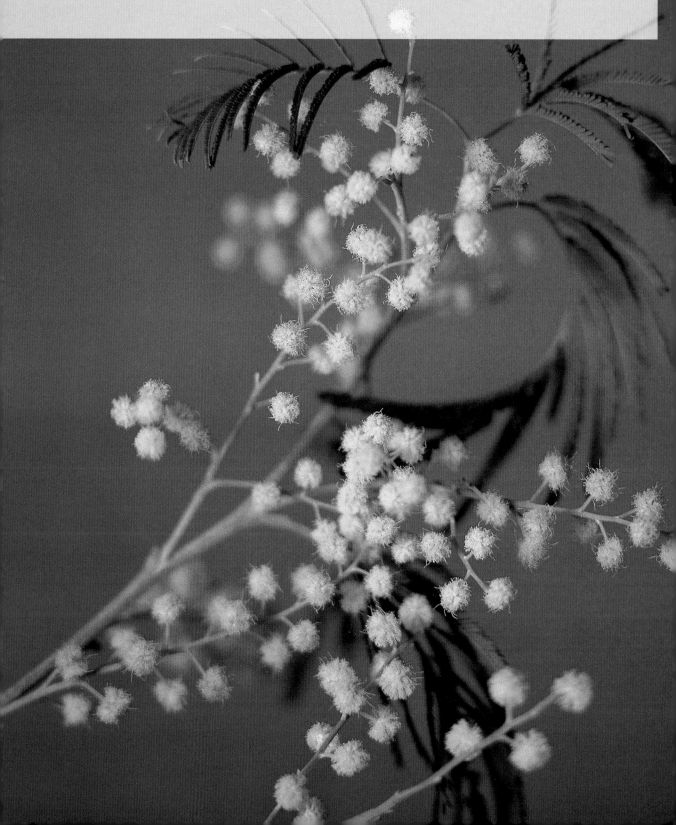

Tip: The Oat Milk Conditioner with Mimosa and Ylang Ylang is a lovely complement to the Chamomile and Geranium Shampoo on page 84.

Conditioners and Rinses

After shampooing, it's important to use conditioner to give increased manageability to your hair, leaving it soft and shiny. Conditioners restore vitality and luster and should be used every time you wash your hair. The following conditioners use essential oils to perfume, balance, and nourish your hair. These homemade conditioners make the perfect complement to your homemade shampoos.

Hair rinses are simple and quick to make, and they are effective in restoring the hair's natural pH balance. Hair rinses are also clarifying and remove any last traces of shampoo or conditioner residue that may remain on the hair shaft. This helps make the hair shine. Use a hair rinse once a week after shampooing and using hair conditioner and make sure you rinse it off thoroughly with a lot of cool or tepid water.

Oat Milk Conditioner with Mimosa and Ylang Ylang

This luxuriant conditioner has a sweet, exotic, and floral fragrance and leaves your hair shiny, soft, and manageable. Oat plant milk softens and nourishes the scalp and hair with its mild, gentle moisturizing properties. Oat milk conditioner is especially good for dry, damaged, and colored hair but is suitable for all hair types.

what's in it?
5 tbsp (75 ml) conditioner base
2 tbsp (25 ml) oat plant milk
10 drops ylang ylang
10 drops lavender
5 drops petitgrain
5 drops mimosa

how's it made?

1 Pour the conditioner base into a glass container with a good pouring spout. Add the oat plant milk and stir thoroughly to combine the all the ingredients.

2 Carefully add the essential oils, one by one. Use a glass stirring rod or a chopstick to thoroughly stir in the oils.

3 Pour into a glass bottle, plastic squeeze bottle, or pump dispenser using a funnel to avoid spillage.

4 Label the bottle and the Oat Milk Conditioner is ready to use.

Herbal Conditioner with Clary Sage and Rosewood

Herbs and rosewood combine to make a conditioner that restores a healthy shine and a fresh, clean smell to your hair. Clary sage helps to reduce excessive production of sebum, especially on the scalp. This conditioner is therefore especially suitable for those who have greasy, lank hair. However, unlike commercial conditioners made for greasy hair, this conditioner actively reduces excessive sebum production, which means your hair stays clean longer.

what's in it?

6½ tbsp (100 ml) conditioner base

10 drops clary sage

10 drops rosewood

5 drops rosemary

3 drops lavender

2 drops tea-tree

how's it made?

1 Pour the conditioner base into a glass container with a good pouring spout.

2 Carefully add the essential oils, one by one. Use a glass stirring rod or a chopstick to thoroughly stir in the oils.

3 Pour into a glass bottle, plastic squeeze bottle, or pump dispenser using a funnel to avoid spillage.

4 Label the bottle and the herbal conditioner is ready to use.

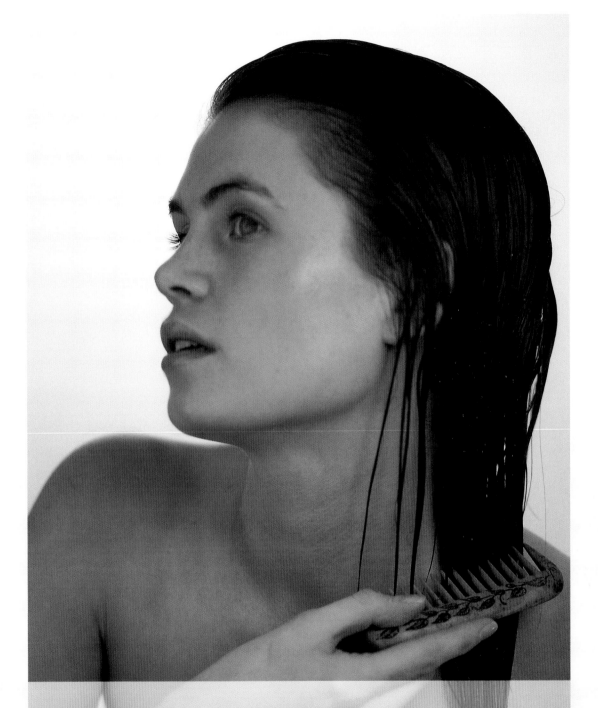

Tip: *Herbal Conditioner with Clary Sage and Rosewood helps reduce excessive sebum production. Massage your scalp vigorously with the conditioner before rinsing it off.*

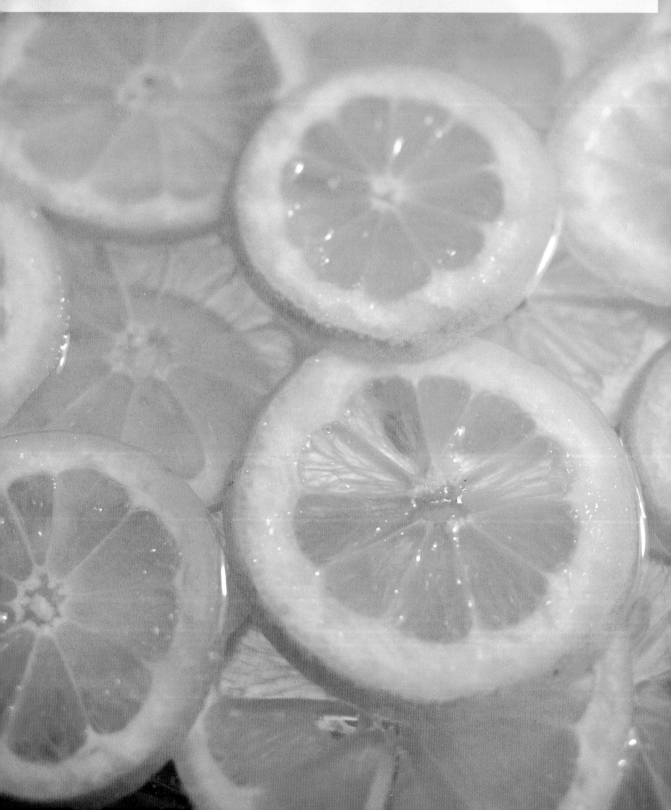

Did You Know? *Lemon has traditionally been used as a hair rinse to brighten dull hair. Its astringent properties also help tone the scalp.*

Apple Cider Vinegar Hair Rinse

Cider vinegar has been used as a hair rinse since the time of our grandmothers, and here apple cider vinegar is used as the base ingredient. Combined with the fresh aroma of orange flower water and petitgrain, this makes a stimulating, clarifying hair rinse. Apple cider vinegar hair rinse is suitable for all hair types, though it works especially well on greasy hair.

what's in it?

1 tsp (5 ml) apple cider vinegar

1 tbsp (10 ml) orange flower water

1 tbsp (10 ml) spring water

3 drops petitgrain

1 drop bergamot

how's it made?

1 Measure the apple cider vinegar into a glass bottle. Add the orange flower water and the spring water. Shake well to combine.

2 Carefully add the essential oils, one by one, and shake well to disperse them.

3 The rinse is ready to use. Slowly pour through your freshly shampooed and conditioned hair. Leave on hair for a couple of minutes.

4 Rinse your hair thoroughly with cool or tepid water.

Lemon and Rosemary Hair Rinse

This recipe uses fresh herbs and lemons—you can easily find fresh organic herbs and citrus fruits. The recipe suggests using rosemary, which is best for dark hair. If you have light hair, substitute chamomile for the rosemary. Parsley is another alternative, and gives your hair a really clean shine.

what's in it?

The juice of one freshly squeezed lemon

1 tsp (5 gm) fresh, finely chopped rosemary, chamomile, or parsley

Enough water to cover the herbs in a small saucepan

how's it made?

1 Squeeze the lemon juice into a glass jug. Put the finely chopped herbs into a saucepan and pour in enough water to cover. Bring to the boil and simmer for five minutes.

2 Strain the mixture through muslin and let the herb infusion cool. Mix 2 tbsp (20 ml) of the herbal infusion into the lemon juice.

3 The rinse is now ready to use. Slowly pour through your freshly shampooed and conditioned hair. Leave on hair for a couple of minutes.

4 Rinse your hair thoroughly with cool or tepid water.

Hot Oil Nourishing Hair Wrap

This treatment is a real treat for your hair. Try to do the hot oil hair wrap once a month. You do need to put aside an evening, but you could combine doing the hair wrap with a body scrub, pedicure, or other beauty treatment. The recipe suggests using almond oil and chamomile, but you can vary the base oil and essential oil according to your hair color and type. Rosemary is good for dark hair. Jojoba oil is good for very dry hair. Sandalwood imparts a lovely, long lasting fragrance, which might be nice for a special occasion.

what's in it?

1 tsp to 1 tbsp (5 to 10 ml) almond oil, depending on
   your hair's length and thickness

3 drops chamomile

how's it made?

1 Warm the almond oil in a small cup or bowl sitting in a larger bowl of hot water. Mix the chamomile in thoroughly.

2 Apply the oil to your hair, making sure you cover every strand. Use the opportunity to give yourself a scalp massage.

3 Wrap your hair in plastic wrap and then cover your head with a hot towel. Replace with another hot towel once the first one has cooled. Leave the oil in for at least two hours.

4 Shampoo your hair at least twice to wash off the oil, then condition your hair as usual. Your hair will feel soft and glossy with a lovely shine.

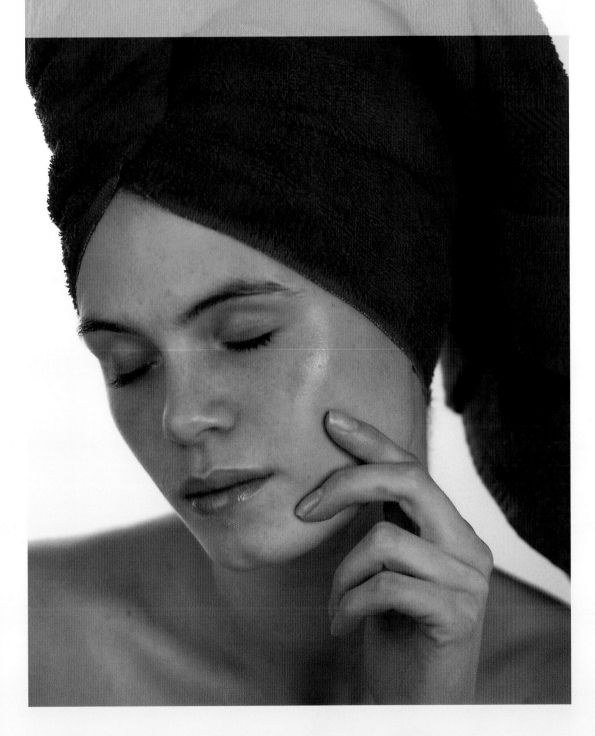

Did You Know? *In India, both men and women routinely use coconut oil as a hair dressing, as it helps protect the hair from the hot sun.*

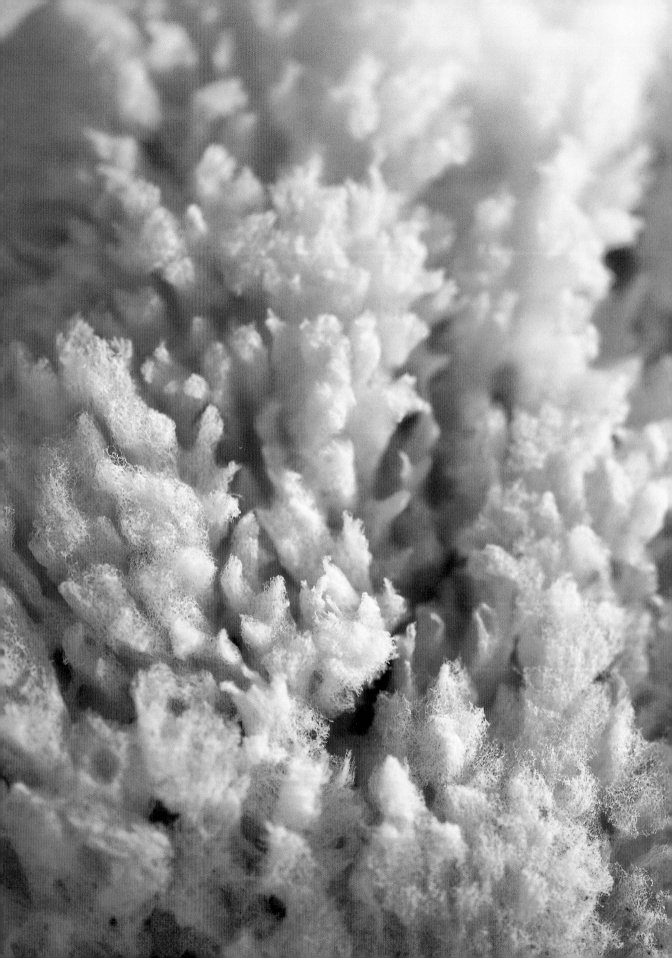

Chapter 6

Naturally Fresh and Clean

"Several essential oils are effective deodorizing agents."
–Patricia Davis, *author and aromatherapist*

Deodorants, Mouthwashes, and Aftershaves

This chapter includes recipes for homemade deodorants, mouthwashes, aftershaves, eye washes, and eye compresses. The recipes are quick and simple to make and lovely to use. All the recipes use only plant-based, natural, and organic ingredients. Essential oils and herbs impart their healing qualities to these cosmetics, and you can rest assured that you are using pure ingredients to keep yourself naturally fresh and clean.

The homemade deodorants have a lovely, clean, fresh aroma. Because they are so gentle on your skin, you can spray them on liberally with no adverse side effects. They will not stain your clothes unlike some commercial deodorants, which can leave white patches on dark clothes or discolor pale-colored ones. The refreshing, uplifting scent will leave you feeling sparkling clean.

However, these homemade deodorants are not as effective or long lasting as many store-bought deodorants. This is because they do not contain any antiperspirant, a substance that actively prevents you from sweating. Our bodies need to sweat, as this is one of the body's ways of cooling down. Sweating also eliminates toxins from the body, so it is a necessary function and should not be discouraged.

The mouthwashes use natural ingredients and essential oils to leave your mouth and gums feeling really fresh and clean. The essential oils also help prevent bacterial growth and discourage and heal mouth ulcers, gum infections, and inflammations such as gingivitis. Using these natural mouthwashes also helps prevent these conditions from arising in the first place and keeps the mouth and gums clean and healthy.

Homemade aftershaves not only are lovely to use but make great gifts for the men in your life. Aftershaves tone the skin after shaving, help reduce redness and skin irritation, and close the pores. Choosing the essential oils you use in your aftershaves means you can not only customize the fragrance to your preference but you can also choose oils that are helpful for the condition of the skin. For instance, a young man just beginning to shave may have acne or delicate skin, and you can choose essential oils to treat both these skin conditions.

Eye washes and eye compresses provide a wonderful relief for tired, red, or itchy eyes. Regular use of these natural homemade remedies can also help prevent eye conditions, such as conjunctivitis, from arising. It is important to remember that you must never put essential oils near, or in, the eyes themselves. These homemade eye washes and eye compresses use herbal infusions and flower waters rather than essential oils and are gentle enough to use on the eyes.

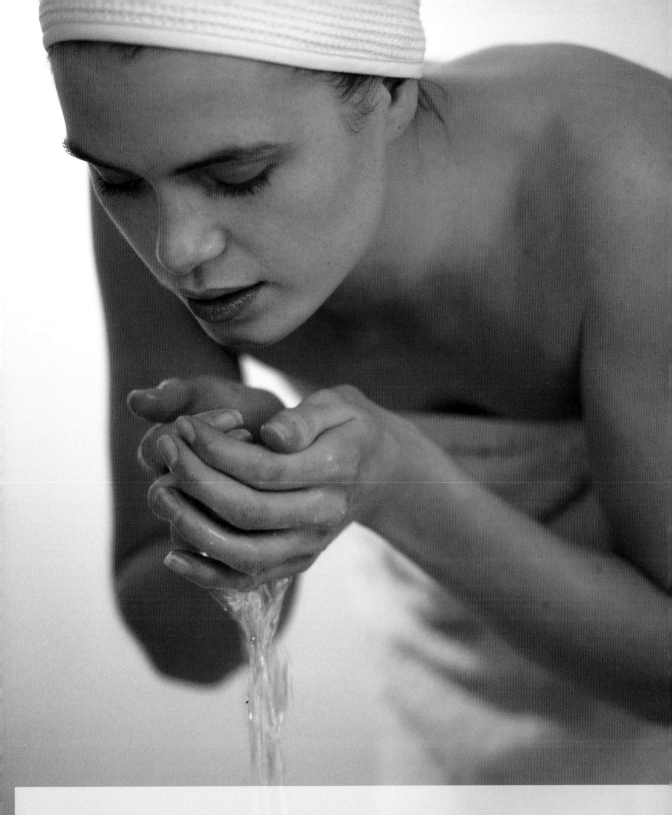

Tip: *Using your homemade deodorants means you may need to wash under your arms a little more frequently, and reapply the deodorant more often—a small price to pay for deodorizing your body naturally.*

Tip: *If you suffer from sweaty feet, you can use this deodorant on your feet as well as under your arms, as the cypress helps prevent excessive sweating.*

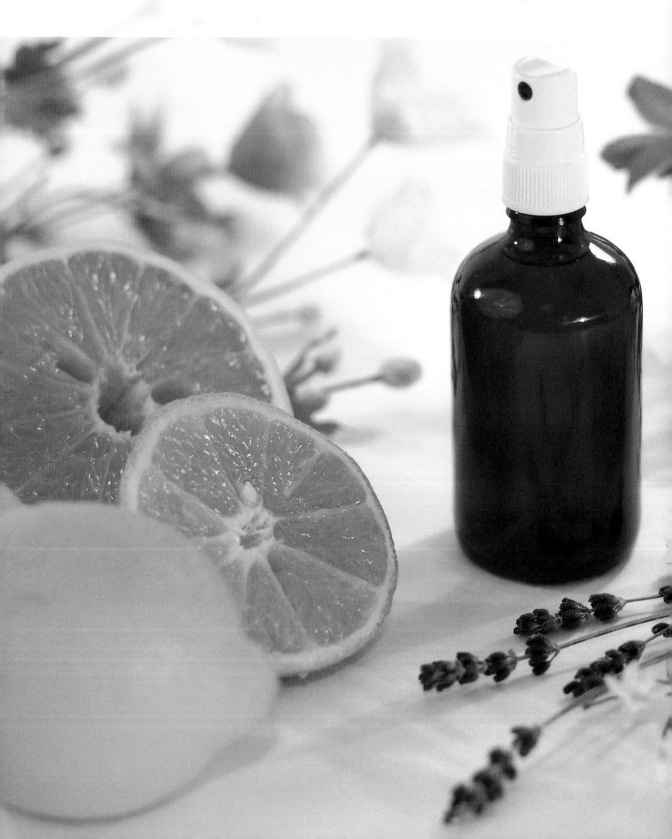

Deodorants

A *quick look at the history of deodorants and perfumes reveals that personal hygiene arrived later than the fragrancing of personal objects, such as gloves, bed linens, and clothes. Indeed, until modern sanitary ware was invented, washing was considered a bit of a nuisance rather than the daily necessity we now take for granted.*

This means that deodorants and perfumes were used to mask body odors, which is still the role of deodorants today. However, by using the following homemade deodorants, you are only applying natural, plant-based ingredients to your body. These work in harmony with your skin and body, keeping you naturally fresh and clean.

Geranium and Cypress Deodorant

This is a classic combination of essential oils with deodorant properties. Geranium is used in skin-care products for its delightful, sweet floral perfume and its astringent and antiseptic properties. Cypress helps reduce excessive sweating, and its fine, woody smell enhances this deodorant. The classic fragrance is deeply refreshing with hints of floral, citrus, and wood, and is suitable for both women and men.

what's in it?

1 tsp high proof vodka

10 drops geranium

10 drops cypress

8 drops bergamot

5 drops neroli

4 drops lavender

3 drops black pepper

4 tbsp (40 ml) witch hazel

2 tbsp (25 ml) cornflower water

2 tbsp (25 ml) orange flower water

how's it made?

1 Measure the vodka into a 4 oz (100 ml) glass bottle with a spray attachment. Carefully add the essential oils, one by one. Shake vigorously to dissolve the essential oils.

2 Pour the witch hazel into the bottle, using a funnel if necessary, followed by the two flower waters. Shake well.

3 Label the bottle and the deodorant is now ready to use.

4 Before you use the deodorant each time, give the bottle a good shake to ensure the essential oils are fully dispersed.

Citrus and Herbal Deodorant

This gentle, antibacterial deodorant uses some of the most effective deodorant essential oils, including bergamot, thyme, and clary sage. Blended with flower waters and witch hazel into a refreshing spray, this deodorant has a delicious, refreshing aroma that is suitable for both women and men.

what's in it?

1 tsp high proof vodka

10 drops bergamot

8 drops clary sage

7 drops thyme

5 drops rosewood

5 drops lemon

3 drops lavender

2 drops mandarin

4 tbsp (40 ml) witch hazel

2 tbsp (25 ml) linden flower water

2 tbsp (25 ml) orange flower water

how's it made?

1 Measure the vodka into a 4 oz (100 ml) glass bottle with a spray attachment. Carefully add the essential oils, one by one. Shake vigorously to dissolve the essential oils.

2 Pour the witch hazel into the bottle, using a funnel if necessary, followed by the two flower waters. Shake well.

3 Label the bottle and the deodorant is now ready to use.

4 Before you use the deodorant each time, give the bottle a good shake to ensure the essential oils are fully dispersed.

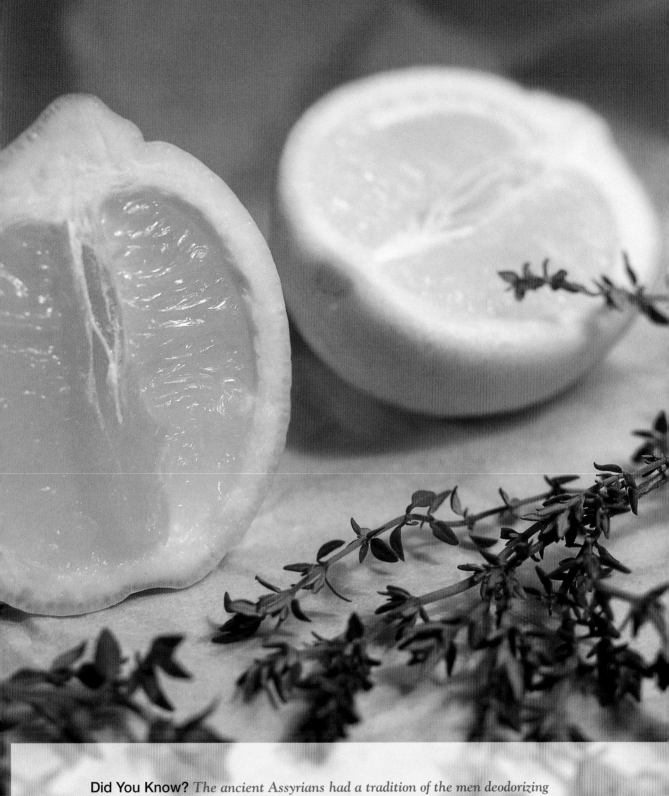

Did You Know? *The ancient Assyrians had a tradition of the men deodorizing their beards.*

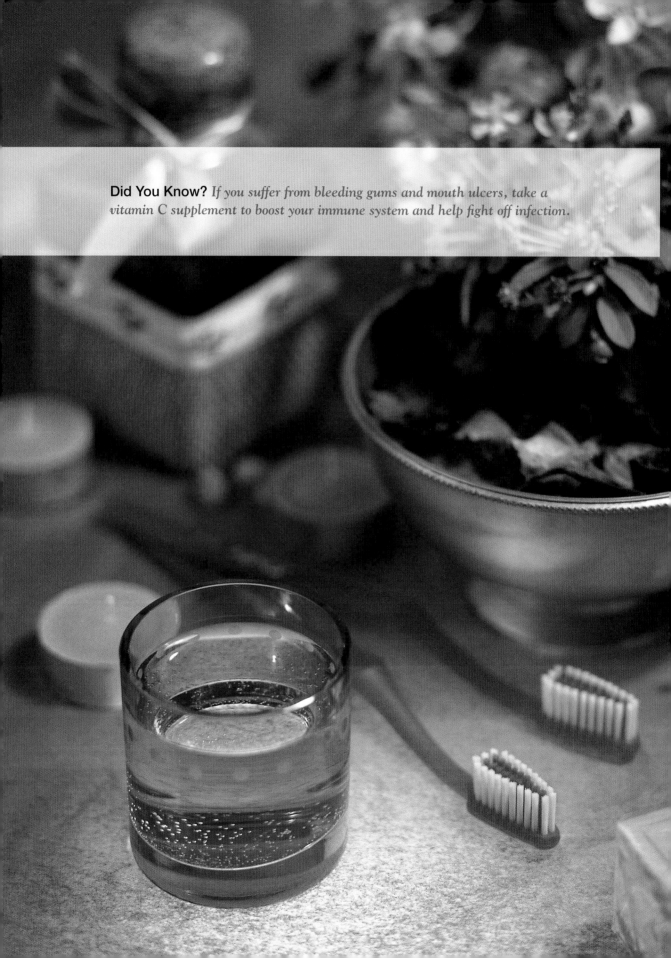

Did You Know? *If you suffer from bleeding gums and mouth ulcers, take a vitamin C supplement to boost your immune system and help fight off infection.*

Mouthwashes

Using a mouthwash daily helps keep your gums healthy and your breath smelling fresh. This daily ritual also helps prevent the build up of plaque on your teeth. Alongside the regular brushing of your teeth with toothpaste and flossing between the teeth, gargles and mouthwashes form an essential part of your daily mouth hygiene routine.

Certain essential oils are very effective in keeping your gums in tip-top condition. Myrrh is traditionally used in toothpastes and mouthwashes as it quickly heals gum disorders and heals mouth ulcers. Fennel is also recommended for use in gargles and mouthwashes as it helps clear gum infections and keeps the mouth smelling fresh and sweet. Alongside peppermint, fennel helps counteract the bitterness of myrrh.

As the following two mouthwashes contain essential oils, remember to spit them out after rinsing your mouth.

Myrrh and Mint Mouthwash

This mouthwash is especially effective if you are having trouble with your gums bleeding or you tend to develop mouth ulcers. The action of the mouthwash is reinforced by using tincture of myrrh as a direct topical application. Put a drop or two of tincture of myrrh on your fingertip and rub over the affected area. It will sting briefly and taste very bitter but the healing effect is well worth it.

how's it made?

1 Pour the brandy or vodka into a 4 oz (100 ml) glass bottle. Carefully add the essential oils one by one. Shake the bottle vigorously to dissolve the oils.

2 Label the bottle and the mouthwash is ready to use. To make one dose of mouthwash, add two or three teaspoons of mouthwash to half a small glass of warm water and stir well.

what's in it?

6 tbsp (90 ml) high proof brandy or vodka

10 drops myrrh

10 drops peppermint

2 drops lemon

1 drop thyme

Fennel Fresh Mouthwash

The clean, fresh, herbal aroma of fennel is balanced with the fruity zing of grapefruit in this tangy mouthwash. Fennel also has a slight aniseed flavor, making it pleasant to use in a mouthwash as well as keeping your mouth and gums clean and healthy.

what's in it?

6 tbsp (90 ml) high proof brandy or vodka

10 drops fennel

10 drops grapefruit

2 drops thyme

1 drop chamomile

how's it made?

1 Pour the brandy or vodka into a 4 oz (100 ml) glass bottle. Carefully add the essential oils, one by one. Shake the bottle vigorously to dissolve the oils.

2 Label the bottle and the mouthwash is ready to use. To make one dose of mouthwash, add two or three teaspoons of mouthwash to half a small glass of warm water and stir well.

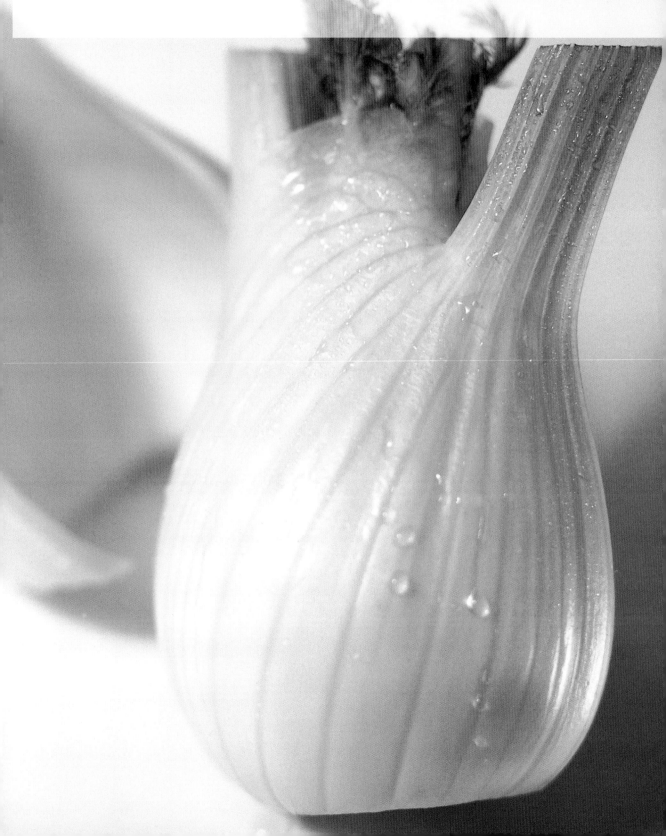

Did You Know? *More people lose their teeth from gum disease than from bad teeth, so looking after your gums is very important.*

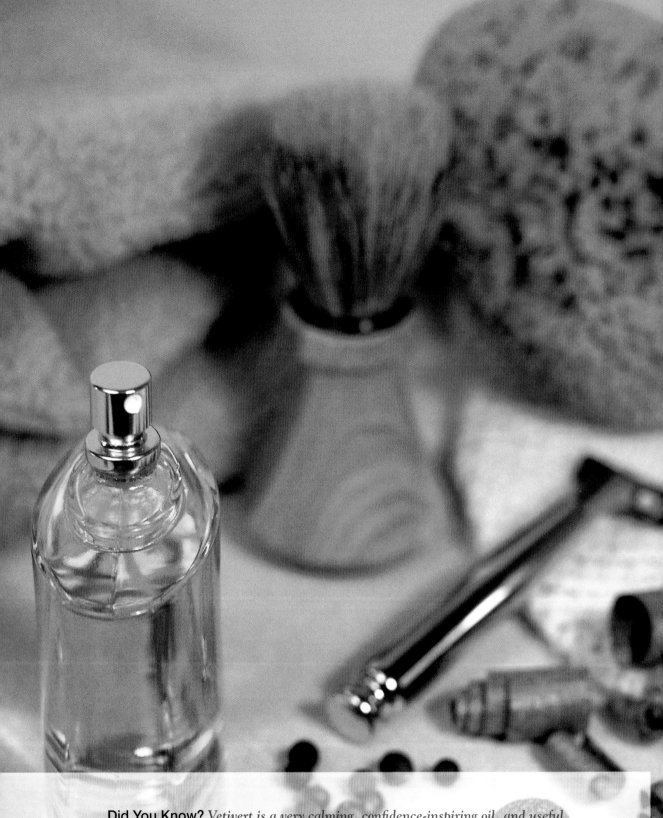

Did You Know? *Vetivert is a very calming, confidence-inspiring oil, and useful for dreamy or overintellectual people.*

Aftershaves

These homemade aftershaves are particularly good for men with sensitive skin and for young men just starting to shave. They are effective but very gentle and help control and prevent razor burn. There are plenty of woody and masculine smelling essential oils that are acceptable to even the most masculine tastes.

Many commercial aftershaves have sickly, cloying, or overpowering scents. The aftershave recipes included here are perfumed only with pure essential oils, and provide more subtle, pleasing, and delicate fragrances. In addition, they tone the skin and close the pores, keeping the skin in good condition.

Sandalwood and Vetivert Aftershave

The sweet, woody, and musky aroma of sandalwood is a particular favorite in aftershaves. Sandalwood is a natural bactericide and soothes the skin after shaving. Vetivert has a deep, earthy aroma that blends beautifully with the sandalwood, creating a strong, deep male fragrance. This aftershave is suitable for all skin types and is particularly good for young men just beginning to shave.

what's in it?

1½ tbsp (20 ml) high proof vodka

8 drops sandalwood

6 drops vetivert

3 drops neroli

4 tbsp (50 ml) witch hazel

6½ tbsp (100 ml) rose water

how's it made?

1 Pour the vodka into a 7 oz (200 ml) glass bottle. Carefully add the essential oils, one by one, and shake vigorously until the oils have dissolved.

2 Add the witch hazel and shake well. Then add the rose water and shake again.

3 Label the bottle and the Sandalwood and Vetivert Aftershave is ready to use.

4 Make sure to shake the bottle before using each time to disperse the oils.

Cedarwood and Juniper Aftershave

Out of all the essential oils, cedarwood is the most popular amongst men, and is much used in men's toiletries. The astringent and antiseptic properties of cedarwood, together with its masculine aroma, make it an obvious choice for a homemade aftershave. Cypress and juniper complement the cedarwood, creating a deep woody fragrance.

what's in it?

1½ tbsp (20 ml) high proof vodka

8 drops cedarwood

6 drops cypress

3 drops juniper

4 tbsp (50 ml) witch hazel

6½ tbsp (100 ml) orange flower water

how's it made?

1 Pour the vodka into a 7 oz (200 ml) glass bottle. Carefully add the essential oils, one by one, and shake vigorously until the oils have dissolved.

2 Add the witch hazel and shake well. Then add the orange flower water and shake again.

3 Label the bottle and the aftershave is ready to use.

4 Make sure to shake the bottle before using each time to disperse the oils.

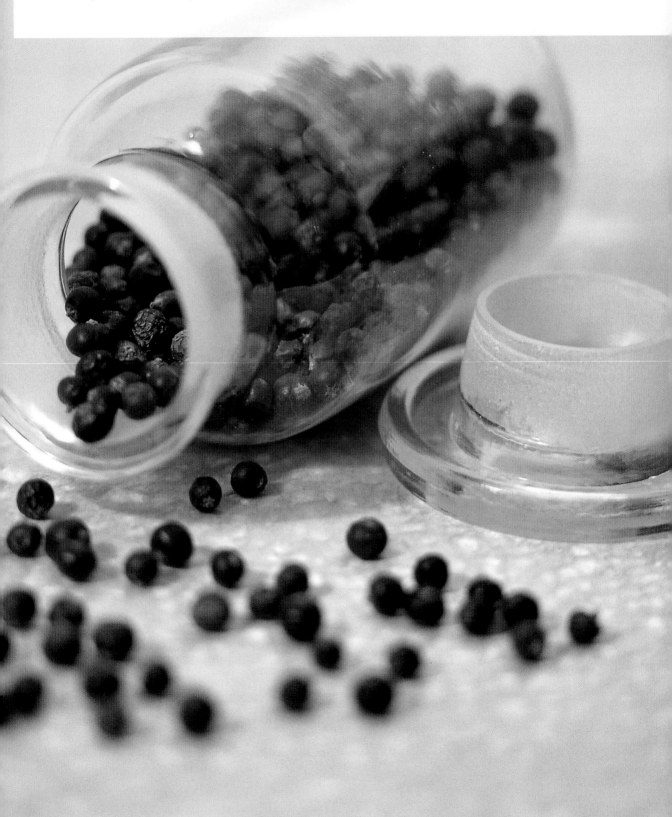

Did You Know? *The popularity of using juniper in men's toiletries is due in part to its cooling and refreshing qualities.*

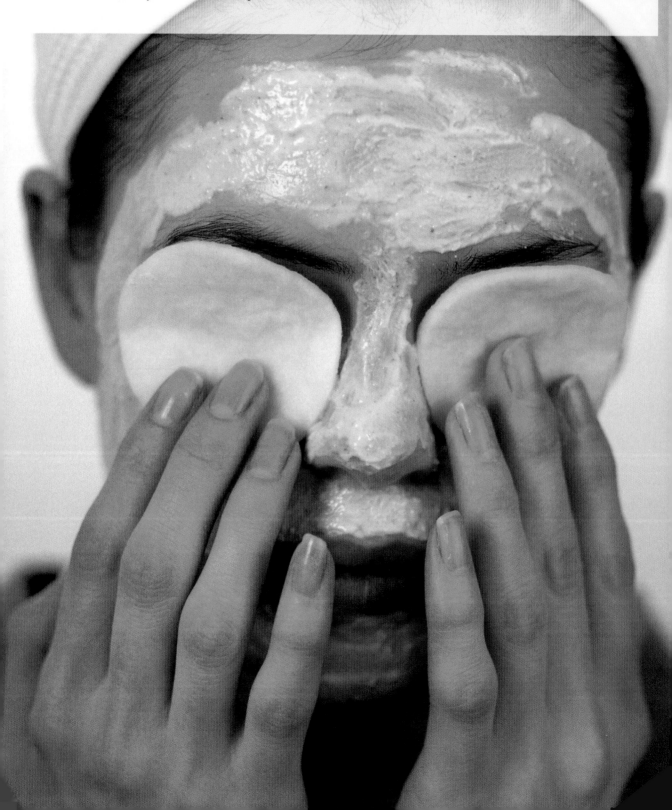

Tip: Eye infections are very contagious. If you have only one eye that is affected, make sure you use a fresh application of the eyewash on the unaffected eye. In fact, it is good practice to use a fresh application for each eye as a standard procedure.

Eye Washes and Compresses

Whenever your eyes are tired, red, and itchy, or you have a mild eye infection such as conjunctivitis, then eye washes and eye compresses made from herbal infusions and flower waters can relieve the symptoms naturally. The recipes that follow use easily obtainable ingredients to make simple remedies. However, if you are short of time or desperate, simply washing the eyes with rose water followed by compresses of used, cooled chamomile tea bags can be effective.

An alternative is to use a homeopathic remedy called euphrasia. This is available both as a liquid and as tablets. Use three to four drops of the liquid in cooled boiled water and rinse the eyes with it. Take tablets as recommended by a homeopath.

Chamomile and Eyebright Eye Wash

Using an infusion of organic chamomile blended with cornflower water makes a cooling, refreshing, and healing eye wash. The addition of tincture of eyebright reinforces the healing action, leaving your eyes refreshed and cooled. There is a long tradition of using cornflower water to wash and refresh the eyes.

what's in it?
1 organic chamomile tea bag
Boiling water to infuse the tea bag
1 tbsp (10 ml) cornflower water
4 drops tincture of eyebright

how's it made?

1 Make an infusion of chamomile as you would make an ordinary cup of tea. Leave it to steep for fifteen minutes.

2 Measure out 1 tbsp (10 ml) of chamomile infusion—you can drink the rest of the tea—and pour it into a 1 oz (25 ml) glass bottle.

3 Add the cornflower water and shake well. Add the eyebright tincture and again shake well.

4 The eye wash is ready to use. Wash each eye with approximately half the quantity of eye wash, as you need to make a fresh batch each time.

Rose Water and Elderflower
Eye Compresses

These cooling, refreshing eye compresses can be used whenever you have ten or fifteen minutes to rest somewhere quietly with your eyes closed. They are effective for eyes that are stinging as a result of air pollution in cities and built up urban areas. You can use the compresses after an eye wash or on their own.

what's in it?
2 drops tincture of elderflower

1 tbsp (10 ml) rose water

2 cotton pads

how's it made?

1 Carefully pour the tincture of elderflower into a small bottle and top off with the rose water. Shake well.

2 Soak the cotton pads with the mixture, apply to your closed eyes, and lie back and rest for ten or fifteen minutes.

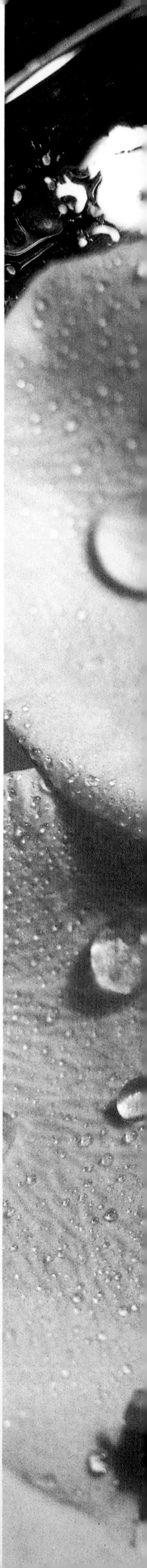

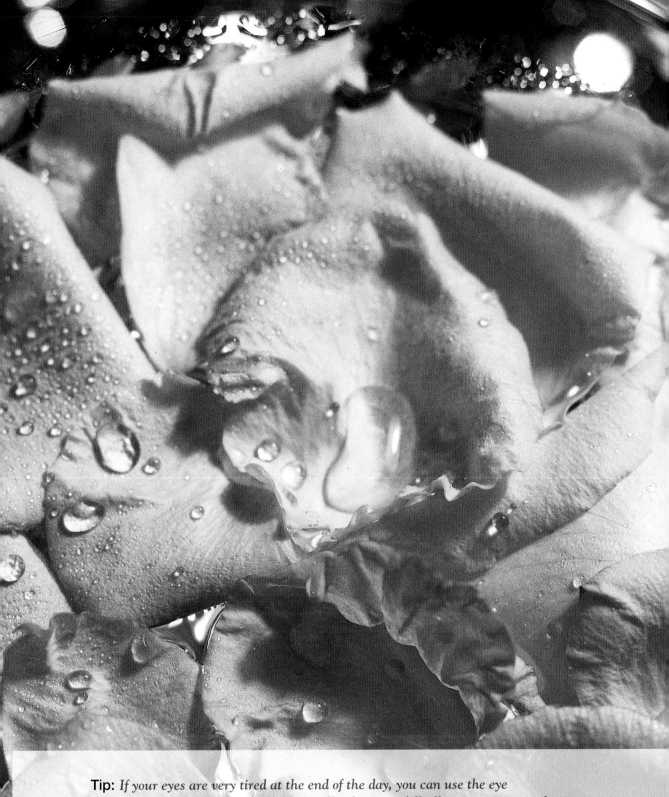

Tip: *If your eyes are very tired at the end of the day, you can use the eye compresses when you go to bed. They will, of course, fall off at some point in the night, but they will have done their work and dried out by then.*

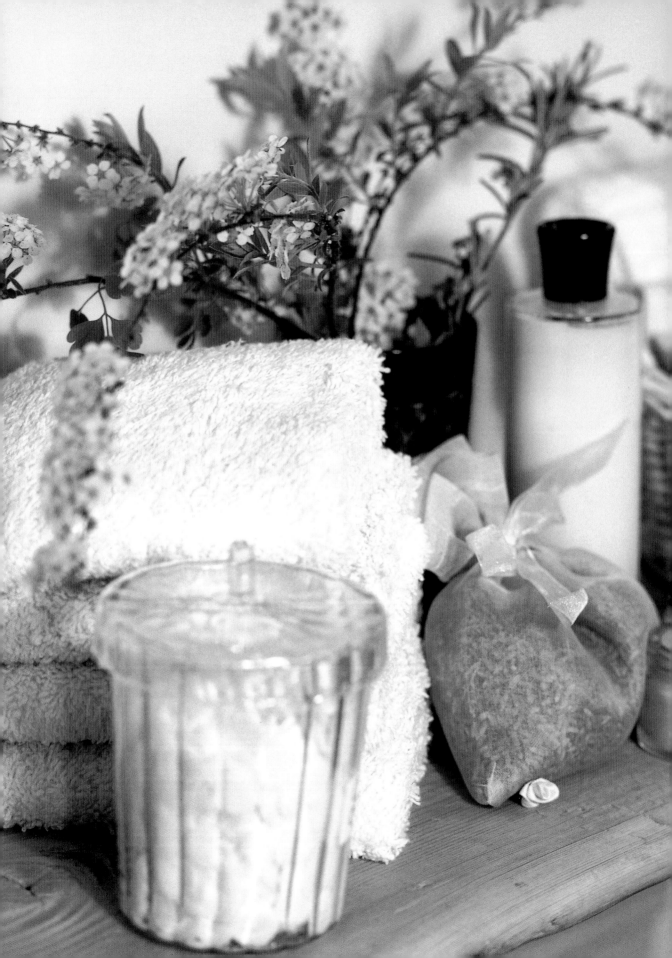

Chapter 7

Gift Wrapping and Storing Your Cosmetics

How To Present Your Cosmetics

Now that you have created some of these wonderful homemade cosmetics, you need some ideas on storing them well. As they make such lovely gifts, some tips on gift wrapping your different homemade creams, lotions, and so forth are also included.

Once your cosmetics have been made, they should be stored carefully. Because they are made from natural, organic ingredients, they do not contain synthetics nor the chemical preservatives found in many store-bought cosmetics. So, although your homemade cosmetics are nice to use, they will not last as long as their store-bought equivalents. This is why the recipes suggest making up quite small quantities: your creams and toners will be used up long before they start to deteriorate.

Another solution to storing your homemade cosmetics is to give some of them away to friends and family! Natural, organic skin- and hair-care products make wonderful health and beauty enhancing gifts, and using some imaginative packaging and presentation ideas can make them look even more attractive. Some of your homemade cosmetics, such as eye washes and face masks, are made to be used immediately and are, unfortunately, not suitable as gifts.

Many of your creams, lotions, lip balms, toners, and aftershaves are kept in glass jars and bottles. You will have noticed that some of the recipes suggest using dark glass while others indicate that clear glass is fine. If you are making cosmetics to give away as gifts—and even to enjoy yourself—try to purchase attractive glass jars and bottles.

With a little effort, you can find pretty-shaped, decorative clear glass bottles, which look much nicer than the plain variety. The most common dark glass jars and bottles are made from amber glass but these can look a bit boring, or even as if they contain medicinal products. A much more attractive option is to seek out dark blue, dark green, and dark red glass jars and bottles. Silver and gold opaque glass jars are also available, which look quite stunning.

Displaying Your Cosmetics

Although your homemade cosmetics need to be kept out of direct sunlight, displaying them attractively on a shelf or on top of a chest of drawers or dressing table can make an attractive room decoration.

A small pyramid of jars makes an eye catching display. Start with three jars on the bottom layer, then two jars on top of those, and finally one jar at the top. Try mixing different colored jars, such as dark blue and silver for a dramatic look.

Take a selection of bottles of toners and lotions and line them up, mixing colors and heights of the bottles. Take an empty bottle, fill it with water, add a small spray of flowers or a single rosebud, and insert in the middle of the line of bottles.

Place folded dark green or blue hand towels and linens on a bathroom shelf, then add bottles and jars of the same color for a coordinated bathroom display.

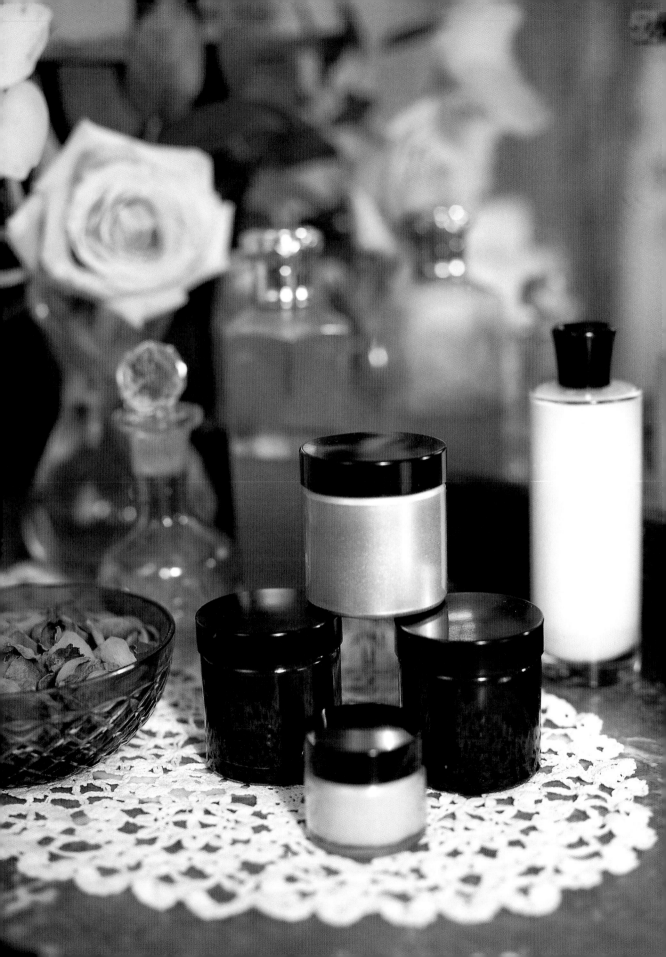

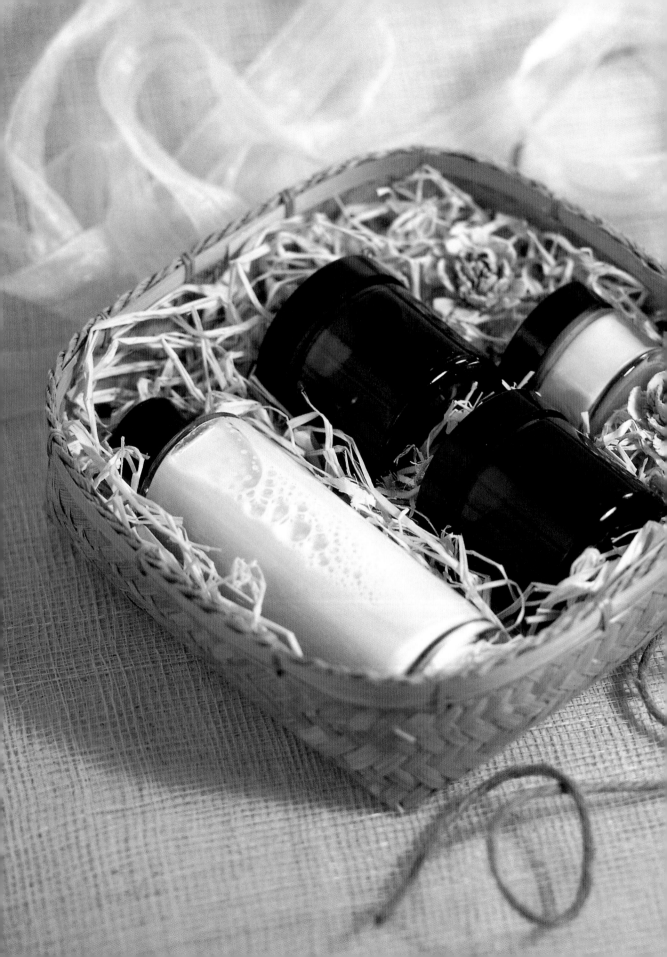

Types of Packaging

Once you have made your lotions and potions, and found attractive glass bottles and jars to put them in, you need to consider how to gift wrap the cosmetics you wish to give away as gifts. The most important point to consider is that glass jars and bottles are fragile, so the packaging must be sturdy enough to protect them adequately and avoid the risk of breakage. Following are some tips for gift wrapping your homemade cosmetics.

Corrugated cardboard is ideal for protecting your jars of face cream and bottles of toner. For bottles, try wrapping a double width length around the bottle twice. Secure with tape, and tie a ribbon, colored string, or strand of raffia around, finishing with a bow. Now fold the open ends closed in a pleat, and either glue them closed or secure them with tape.

Some handcrafted papers are quite stiff and make an attractive alternative to corrugated cardboard. You can fray the ends for a rustic look or cut them with pinking shears.

Colored tissue paper makes an attractive wrapping but is not sufficient on its own to protect glass jars and bottles. Try wrapping a sheet of colored tissue around your jars and bottles, and then wrapping with corrugated cardboard or handcrafted paper.

Boxes—either wood or cardboard—are ideal to package and present your jars and bottles. Try nestling the bottles and jars in shredded paper, raffia, or colored tissue paper. You could also include dried flowers for extra effect.

For a stunning present, take a large wooden box and fill it with a selection of dried flowers and petals. Choose three or four handmade cosmetics that complement each other; a nice combination might include Honey and Rose Lip Balm (page 57), Rose and Geranium skin toner (page 29), Cocoa Butter and Rose Cream (page 41), and Rejuvenating Rose Bath Milk (page 68). Place the different bottles and jars in among the dried flowers and wrap a sheet of clear plastic over the top.

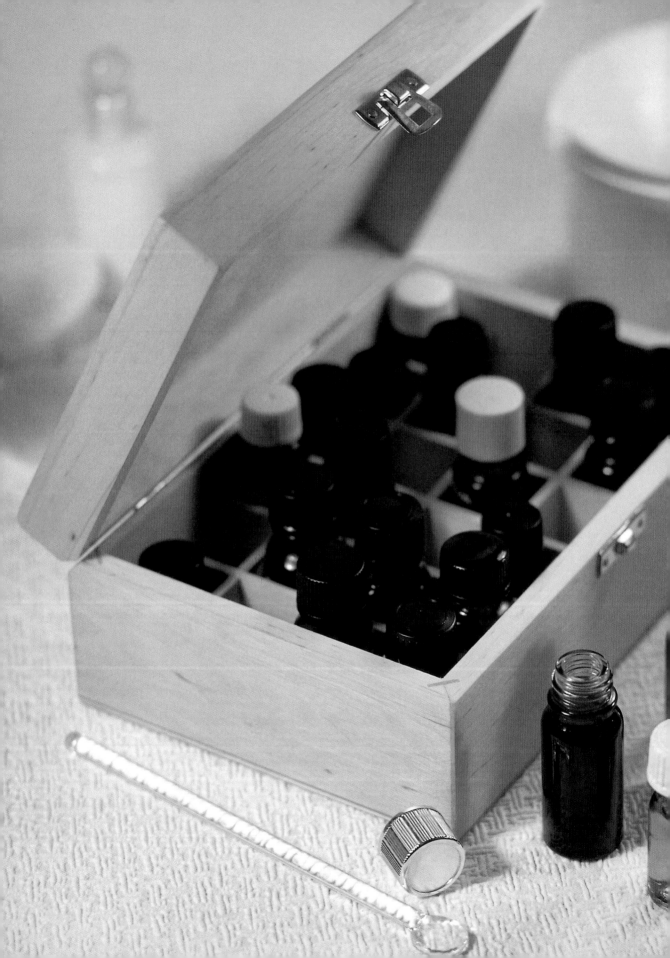

Storing Fresh and Dried Ingredients

Buying and storing all your homemade cosmetic ingredients properly is of fundamental importance to the overall process of making them. The suppliers listed in the directory on the following two pages give you a range of professional suppliers of all the ingredients you will need to successfully make skin creams, lotions, toners, deodorants, shampoos, conditioners, and so forth. Following are some tips on how to store and keep your ingredients properly, and also tips on storing your skin-care products once you've made them.

- All ingredients are best bought fresh. Although the different ingredients for the various cosmetics have differing shelf lives, it is a good habit to buy your ingredients only as you need them.

- Only buy sufficient quantities for your immediate requirements. Even if you can receive a discount for buying larger quantities of ingredients, unless you use it up quickly it could prove a false economy.

- Store your ingredients in a cool, dark, dry place away from drafts, light, damp, and heat. This will help prolong shelf life.

- Make sure you store your bottles of essential oils upright, in a cool dark place.

- Many flower waters are supplied in thick, clear plastic bottles. Transfer them into dark glass bottles as soon as possible. Flower waters only have a limited shelf life, and storing them in dark glass bottles will help prolong this somewhat.

- Fresh ingredients such as yogurt, ground almonds, cucumber, herbs, fruits, and honey should be as fresh as possible, especially for organic produce.

- If you have used half a container of base lotion, cleanser, skin cream, or other base product, consider transferring the remainder to a smaller container. This will prevent too much air from coming into contact with the base ingredient, which could spoil it more rapidly.

- If you think something has gone bad because it has discolored or changed texture, then throw it away and buy new supplies. Using old, imperfect ingredients could affect how a recipe turns out, and you don't want to waste other ingredients.

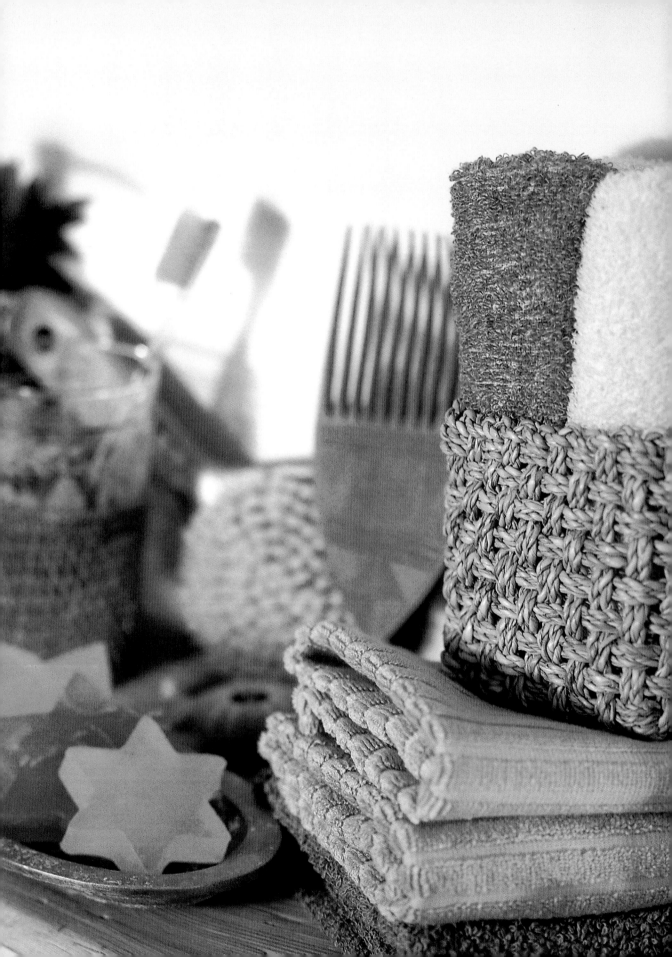

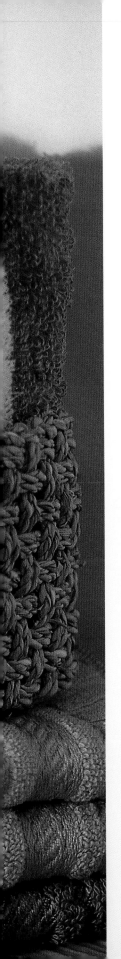

Chapter 8

All About Soap

All About Soap

The quotation on page 119 describes briefly the science of soap, or in other words, how and why soap cleans. You will also discover from the quote that soap is made primarily from fat or oil and caustic soda, which doesn't make soap sound very nice! That is why this book suggests ways of making soaps that are kind to your skin and the environment. By using pure vegetable oils and plant-based colors, essential oils, and other organic nutrients, you can create soaps that look and feel close to nature.

Soap has an interesting history, and according to legend was discovered by accident in ancient Rome. To please their gods, the Romans performed animal sacrifices on Sapo Hill. The women rinsed their clothes in the Tiber River, which runs at the base of Sapo Hill. The women noticed a soapy mix of animal fat and caustic wood ashes seeping into the river. When this came in to contact with their clothes, the dirt on them seemed to magically wash away. After this discovery, soap was made deliberately and proved most popular.

Europeans' interest in washing declined after the fall of the Roman Empire. However, in the seventh century, soap was produced again in limited quantities in Italy, France, and Spain, but only as a luxury item for the wealthy. Therefore, making basic soap at home, from scraps of animal fat, became part of the seasonal cycle of village life.

Early forms of soap were made using animal fat. Today's commercially produced soap is still made with tallow, although all-vegetable soaps are becoming increasingly available. In keeping with the organic ethics of this book, all the included recipes use only vegetable oils.

Animal fats are highly saturated and clog the skin's pores, causing blackheads and other blemishes. Tallow can also cause eczema and allergies in people with sensitive skin. Animal fats are used in soap production however because they are considerably cheaper and easier to use, as they can withstand higher temperatures and are less temperamental than vegetable oils.

Health-food shops and herbal gift shops offer pure, organic, all-vegetable soaps, which, although lovely to use and ethically produced, are quite expensive. When you make your own soap, you use only quality ingredients that are suited to your skin. And after the initial outlay of purchasing basic soap making ingredients, you might even find you'll be saving money on soap.

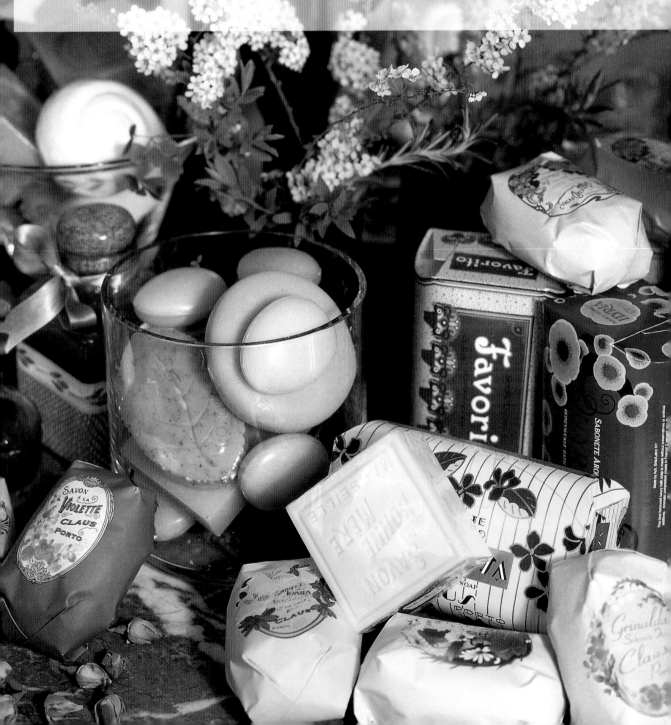

"Soap is a chemical combination of caustic soda and fat or oil. The soap molecule has two ends. One end—the caustic soda—is attracted to water. The other end—the fat or oil—is attracted to grease and dirt. Thus, although they normally don't mix, the soap pulls grease and dirt into solution in water."
—Ian Marshall, doctor, psychotherapist & author

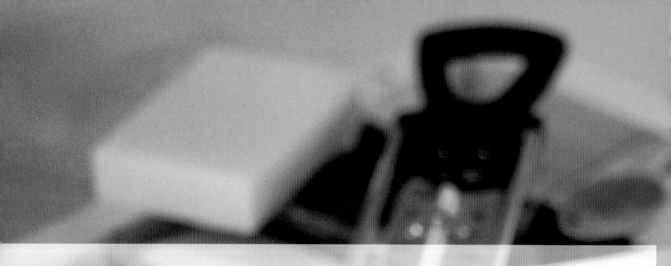

Did You Know? The German chemist Justus von Leibig suggested that much could be learned about a nation by measuring its per capita consumption of soap. Accordingly, those countries that used the most soap were the most civilized.

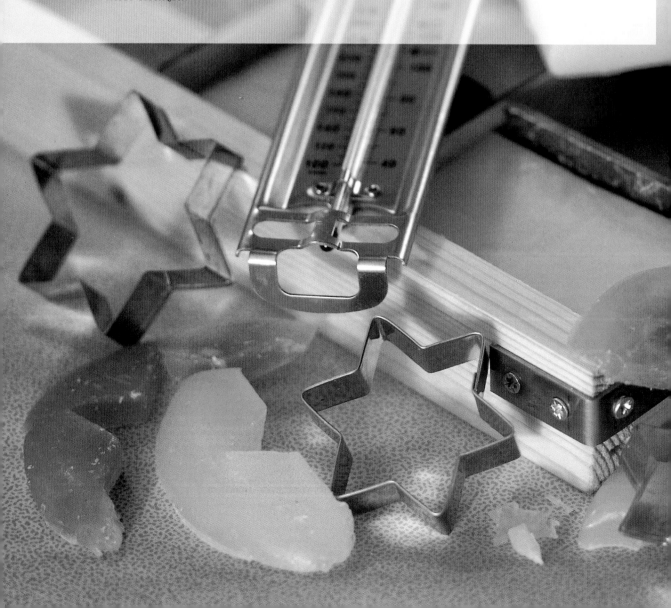

What You Will Need

Most basic soap making equipment can be found in the kitchen, so you probably don't have to buy a lot of extra implements. Make sure you wash all kitchen utensils thoroughly after making soap before using them again for cooking. You will need the following utensils:

- Scales, preferably digital and electronic. Weighing ingredients, even liquids, is more accurate than measuring by volume. Accurate measuring of ingredients—especially for cold-process soaps—is crucial.
- A large, stainless-steel or ceramic saucepan or pot, which is resistant to corrosion from lye, the solution of caustic soda and water. A double boiler is also necessary for some recipes.
- A large, lye-resistant glass bowl
- A cheese grater
- A sharp knife
- A large glass measuring cup and a smaller measuring cup
- An electric beater or hand whisk
- A cooking thermometer
- Rubber gloves and protective eye glasses or goggles—caustic soda and lye can cause nasty burns if they touch the skin, so they must be treated carefully and with respect. Wear the gloves and goggles throughout the entire process when you make cold-process soap.
- A wooden or stainless-steel spoon
- A mortar and pestle
- Soap molds—specially designed soap molds; cookie, jello, or cake molds; small cups and bowls; or even small cardboard boxes. Most recipes make approximately twelve bars of soap in a professional soap mold. If you use jello molds, cups, bowls, etc, then estimate the size of each mold according to a bar of soap, and prepare enough molds before starting.
- Plastic wrap
- Waxed paper
- Cookie cutters are also useful to cut soap into pretty shapes.

Different types of soaps require different ingredients, so it is best to check each recipe beforehand to make sure you know exactly what you will need. The base products and some of the other ingredients need to be purchased from a specialist supplier (see pages 222–223). A list of basic ingredients is below:

- Base oils: coconut, soya bean, light olive oil (not extra virgin)
- Caustic soda (cold-pressed soaps only)
- Soap flakes, liquid soap base, shower gel base, bubble bath base
- Block glycerin
- A range of essential oils
- Herbs, dried flowers, oats, rosehip granules, and spices for natural colors and textures
- Nutrients to enrich the soaps, including shea butter, cocoa butter, almond oil, avocado oil, jojoba oil, rosehip oil, beeswax, Monoi de Tahiti, honey, liquid glycerin.

Basic Techniques

Making cold-process soap is complex, but don't fret. These instructions supplement the individual recipes to give you the best chance of success.

Cold-process soap is based on saponification, meaning a chemical reaction between an acid (oils) and a base (lye). The acid and the base combine to form a syrupy mixture, which is poured into molds to set. Attaining the correct temperature is essential to this process, and the oils and lye must be the same temperature when mixed, between 95°F (35°C) and 100°F (38°C). This is not so simple, because when you add caustic soda to water it heats up to well over 100°F (38°C), so you need to let it cool while you heat the oils.

It is helpful to have a bowl of cold water standing by so you can cool the lye to match the temperature of the oils. Similarly, if the oils heat too much, you can cool them in the same manner.

Add the lye to the oils, pouring slowly and stirring continuously. Be careful to avoid splashing. Once all the lye has been added, keep stirring the mixture until it starts to trace. Tracing occurs when the mixture has become opaque and thick enough to drizzle a pattern on the surface of the soap and not have it sink in. Be careful not to stir too vigorously—which will create air bubbles—but briskly enough to mix the two liquids thoroughly.

Tracing usually occurs between fifteen minutes and a couple of hours, depending on the recipe. Be patient. If tracing hasn't happened after an hour, leave the mixture off the heat and stir it occasionally. If the balance of oils to lye wasn't quite accurate, or if the two were not exactly the same temperature, then tracing may take up to forty-eight hours. If it hasn't happened by then, it won't, so throw the mixture away and start again.

After tracing, you can add essential oils, color, nutrients, and other ingredients to give the soap texture. Make sure ingredients such as dried flowers or oats are finely ground. Also ensure that nutrients such as honey are warmed slightly so the warm, saponified soap mixture isn't "shocked" by adding cold substances.

Once you've added the ingredients and nutrients, prepare the molds by lightly greasing them with oil, making it easy to remove the soap from the molds. Slowly pour the liquid into your molds, cover the molds with plastic wrap or cardboard, place them somewhere warm, and cover with blankets. This ensures the soap cools slowly and allows the saponification process to continue. After twenty-four hours uncover the molds and let them sit for four to seven days.

Check the soap regularly. When it's hard enough to cut and retain its shape, remove it from the mold. If you used a large mold, cut the soap into individual bars. You must still wear rubber gloves, as the saponification is not complete and the caustic could still irritate your skin. Let the soap sit in a warm, dry place for three to four weeks, turning once halfway through. This is the final curing process, during which the soap becomes hard and mild, and is then ready to use.

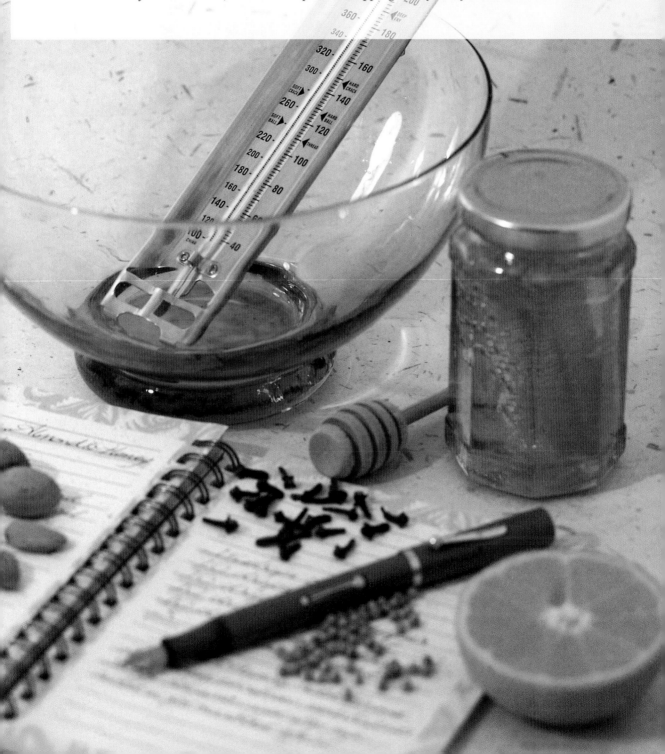

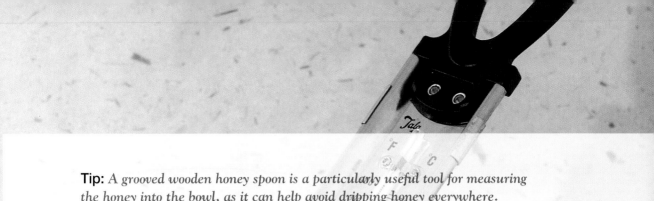

Tip: *A grooved wooden honey spoon is a particularly useful tool for measuring the honey into the bowl, as it can help avoid dripping honey everywhere.*

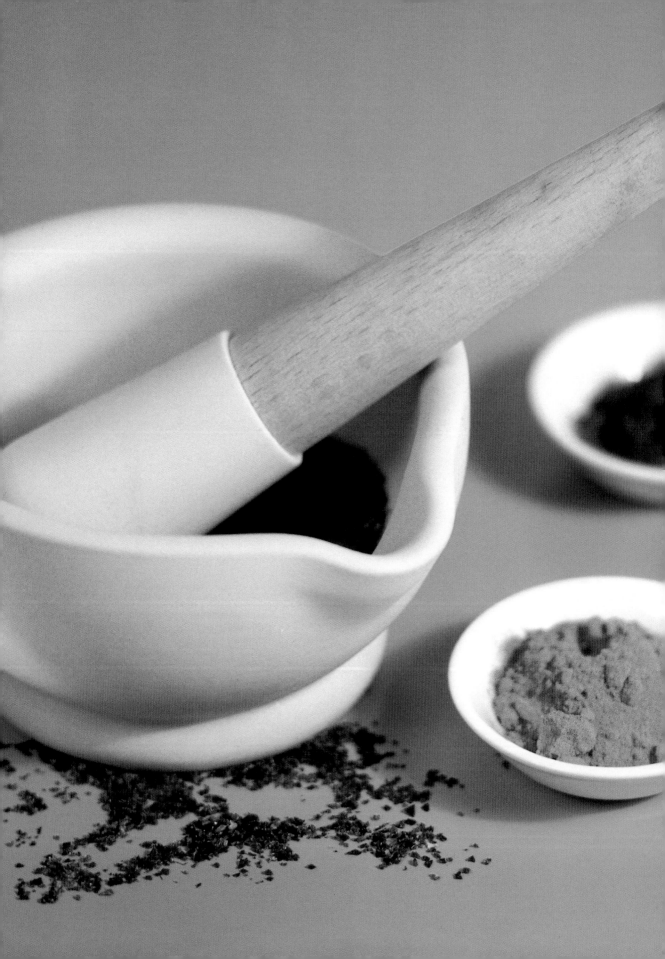

Chapter 9

Natural Colors

Color Your Soaps

There are many different ways to color soaps, but some are artificial and unpleasant. Bright green, vibrant purple, and deep pink soaps are colored with synthetic chemicals, and come with possible health risks. However, it is surprisingly easy to use natural, organic herbs and spices to color your soaps, and a few essential oils give color, too. You will not obtain the bright, uniform colors achieved with synthetics, but instead you will get warm, earthy, unevenly colored, and natural-looking soaps.

On the right is a list of natural ingredients with which to color your soaps. Because you are working with natural and organic substances, there is no guarantee of exact color, but the variations and new discoveries are part of the fun of making your own soaps. With herbs, spices, and roots, make sure they are finely ground. Then stir ½ or 1 teaspoon full into 2 teaspoons of heated vegetable oil. Mix well, and then filter out larger particles with a tea strainer or coffee filter before mixing into the soap. When using essential oils, remember they will also perfume your soaps. First mix in ten drops and, if you want a stronger shade of color, keep adding drops one by one till you get the desired shade.

Color	Ingredient
Yellow	Turmeric
Orange	Turmeric and Paprika
Red/Mauve	Alkanet Root
Pink	Rosehip Granules
Blue	Blue Chamomile or Blue Cypress essential oil
Green	Blue Chamomile and Turmeric
Brown	Cinnamon
Peach	Paprika

These are a few basic ideas to get you started. Don't be afraid to experiment with other natural ingredients, and by varying the quantities of colorant and oil you will achieve different shades, tones, and colors.

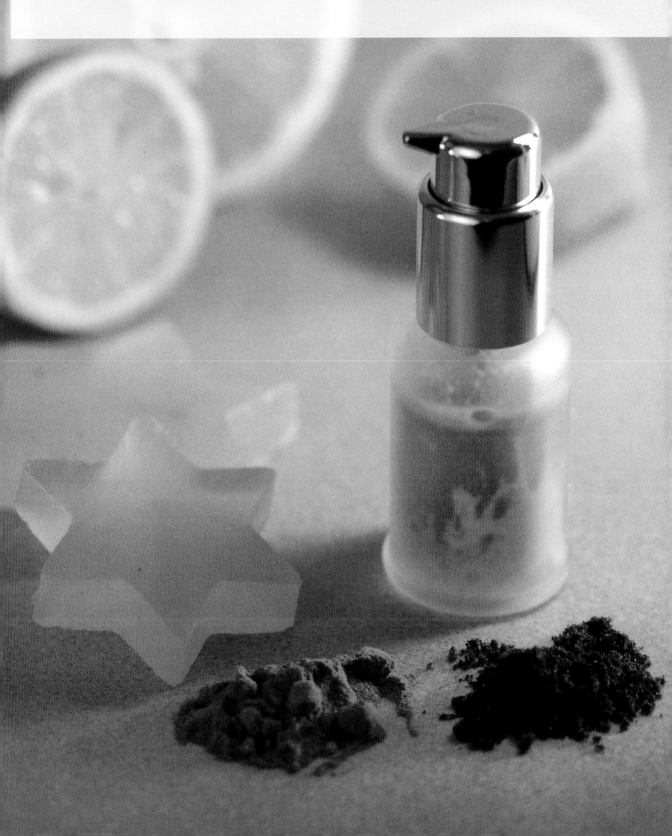

Tip: *Try swirling the color in briefly, rather than mixing it in thoroughly. This will give you an attractive rippled effect rather than a uniformly colored soap.*

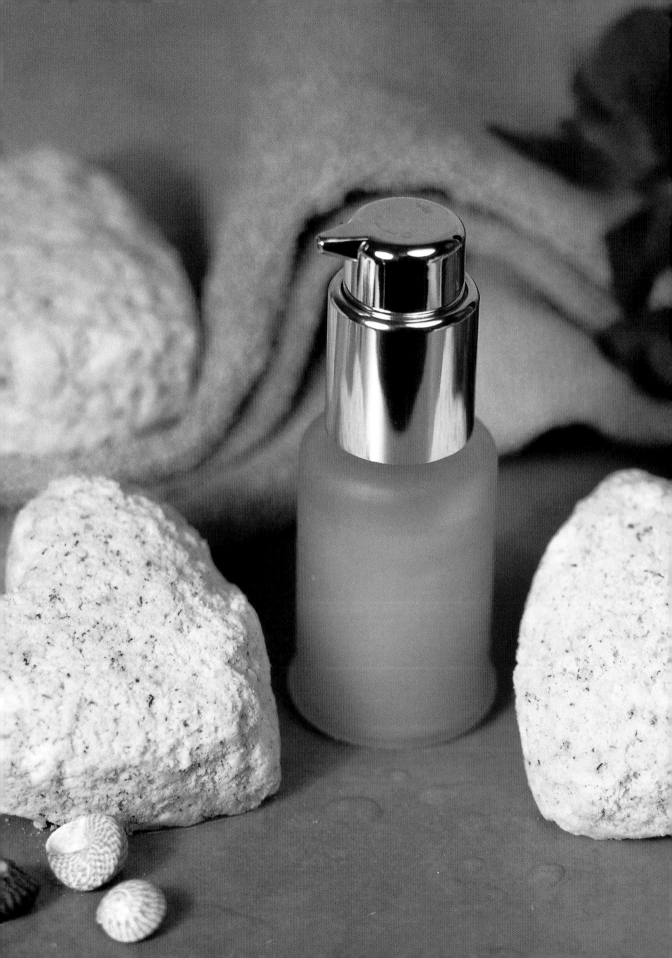

Chapter 10

Liquid Soaps,
Bath Bombs,
Bubble Baths,
and Shower Gels

Getting Started

This chapter contains some really simple recipes to get you started on the soap maker's path. The recipes for liquid soaps, bubble baths, and shower gels require cosmetic base products, which you can easily purchase from the list of specialist suppliers (see pages 222–223). Some stores that offer natural, herbal remedies and essential oils are also beginning to sell a few base products for homemade soaps and cosmetics.

Don't be put off by the long list of strange ingredients in the base products. These are just the proper technical or chemical terms. For example, aqua simply means water.

When purchasing base products, make sure they contain no fragrances and are uncolored. Cosmetic bases should ideally be vegetable oil or water based, so essential oils will mix in easily.

Liquid soaps can be made by simply mixing the base with essential oils and a color base, if desired. You can experiment with your own favorite blends of essential oils and try out different natural colors. Once you feel confident with your experimenting, you can even add a few drops of herbal tinctures to add different healing qualities.

Bath bombs, or bath tablets, make a wonderfully scented and exuberant fizz when they hit water. Easy to make and fun to use, bath bombs bring out the inner child. A key ingredient, baking soda, is more familiar in the kitchen for baking cakes but has traditionally also been used in bathing to calm irritated skin.

Bubble baths and shower gels are made in a similar way to liquid soaps, by simply mixing in essential oils and color. The recipes given here are a good start, but you can also experiment to create your own personalized bathing products.

Make sure you use a large enough container to stir essential oils and colors into the base thoroughly without spilling over. Mix steadily, but not too vigorously; you don't want too many bubbles until the soap or bubble bath is being used.

The best tool for mixing essential oils and colors into the base products is a glass stirring rod. Specially designed for this purpose, you can purchase a glass stirring rod from one of the specialist suppliers listed (see pages 222–223) or a kitchen-supply store. Alternatively, you can use a wooden or plastic chopstick.

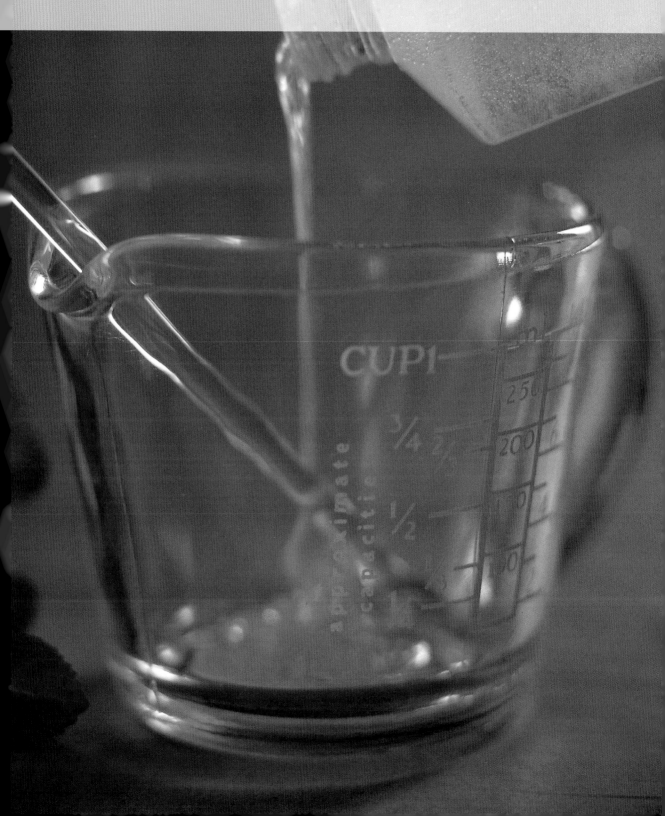

"By purchasing fine-quality essential oils and absolutes, along with natural base products, you will be able to create recipes that are natural, fragrant, gentle, and easy to follow."

–Janita Morris, *author and scent maker*

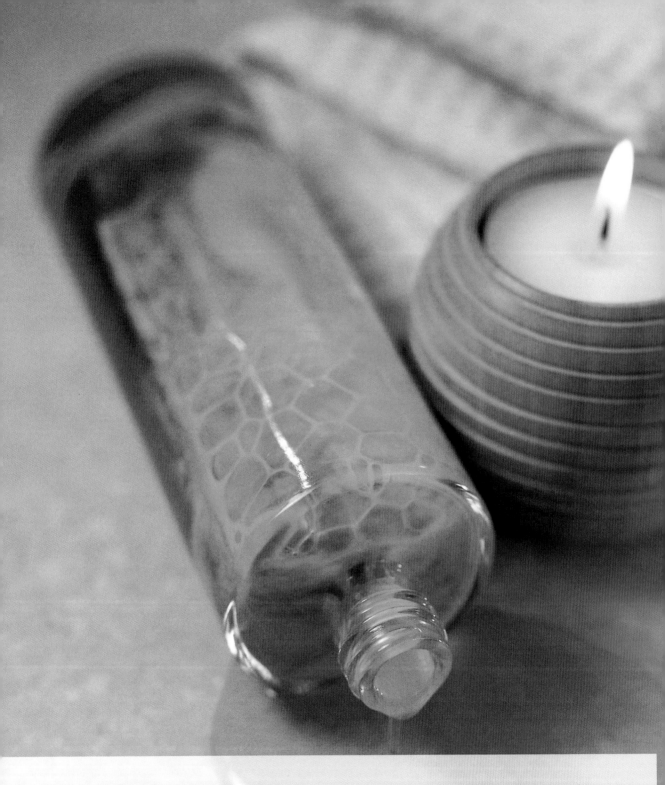

Did You Know? *Citrus essential oils are obtained by a technique called expression, which means simply squeezing the fruit peel to extract the naturally occurring essential oil. This is quite easy to do at home, and you could substitute all or some of the essential oil with some you expressed yourself from fresh, organic citrus fruits.*

Liquid Soaps

Liquid soaps are equally popular in the kitchen and the bathroom. They are most easily used in a pump dispenser bottle. One of the great advantages of liquid soaps in pump dispenser bottles is that they are completely hygienic. Each squirt is fresh and untouched by anyone else, unlike traditional bars of soap, which are handled by every bather. This makes them the best choice for public bathrooms, restaurant kitchens, and other places where hygiene is at a premium.

Liquid soaps are quite a recent innovation, but their popularity and hygienic qualities have ensured that their use is now widespread. The hygienic quality of liquid soaps can be enhanced by the addition of essential oils such as tea tree, a powerful bactericide and antiseptic, although all essential oils are natural antiseptics to some degree. This means that you can make floral and herbal liquid soaps and know that they are effectively antiseptic.

Citrus Suds

The fresh, clean smell of citrus oils is a favorite for cleaning products. Here, the tang of lemon and the warmth of orange combine to make a sweet, fresh scent. This recipe also contains a few drops of sandalwood. This gives the soap a deeper, long-lasting scent. Citrus Suds is colored with orange in the recipe below, but you could substitute yellow if you prefer, or leave it uncolored.

what's in it?

8½ fl oz (250 ml) liquid soap base
12 drops lemon
10 drops orange
4 drops grapefruit
4 drops sandalwood
10 drops orange color (see page 126)

how's it made?

1 Pour the liquid soap into a container that holds at least 16 fl oz (500 ml) and has a good pouring spout.

2 Carefully drop in the essential oils, one by one, followed by the color.

3 Mix thoroughly into the liquid soap base. Be careful not to create too many bubbles.

4 Pour the mixture into a bottle or pump dispenser. The Citrus Suds liquid soap is now ready to use.

Lavender Lather

Lavender has been in popular, continuous use for thousands of years in all its different forms of fresh and dried flowers, essential oil, and lavender water. It is also a prime ingredient of traditional potpourri. One use that may be familiar to many readers is the lavender sachets that are moth repellent and freshening. Our grandmother's generation used to make them each summer and place them in wardrobes and clothes chests. Another traditional use of lavender is to fragrance soap.

what's in it?

8½ fl oz (250 ml) liquid soap base

20 drops lavender

5 drops geranium

5 drops rosemary

how's it made?

1 Pour the liquid soap into a container that holds at least 16 fl oz (500 ml) and has a good pouring spout.

2 Carefully drop in all the essential oils, one by one.

3 Mix thoroughly into the liquid soap base. Be careful not to create too many bubbles.

4 Pour the mixture into a bottle or pump dispenser. The Lavender Lather liquid soap is now ready to use.

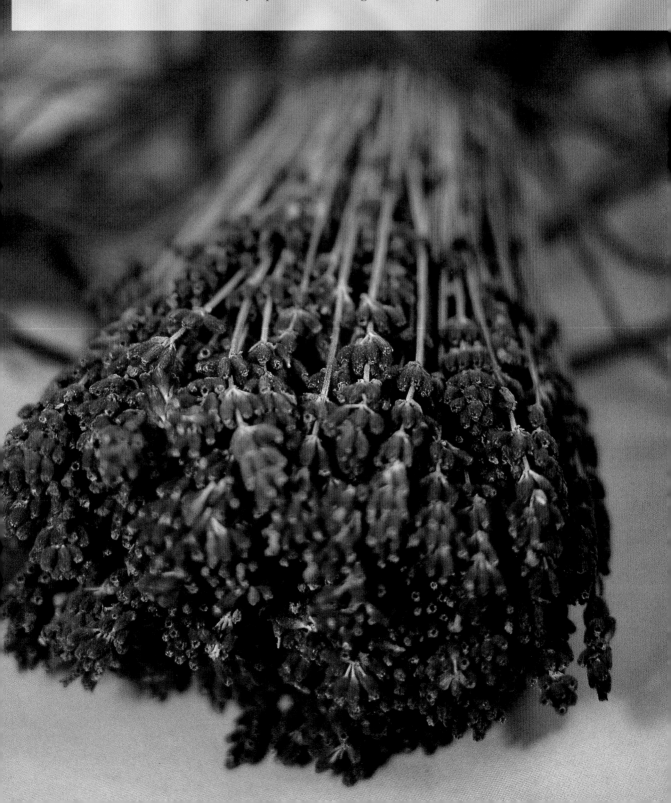

Did You Know? *The name of lavender comes from the Latin word* lavare, *which means "to wash." Lavender is a natural antiseptic and was used to cleanse wounds as well as for personal washing and laundry.*

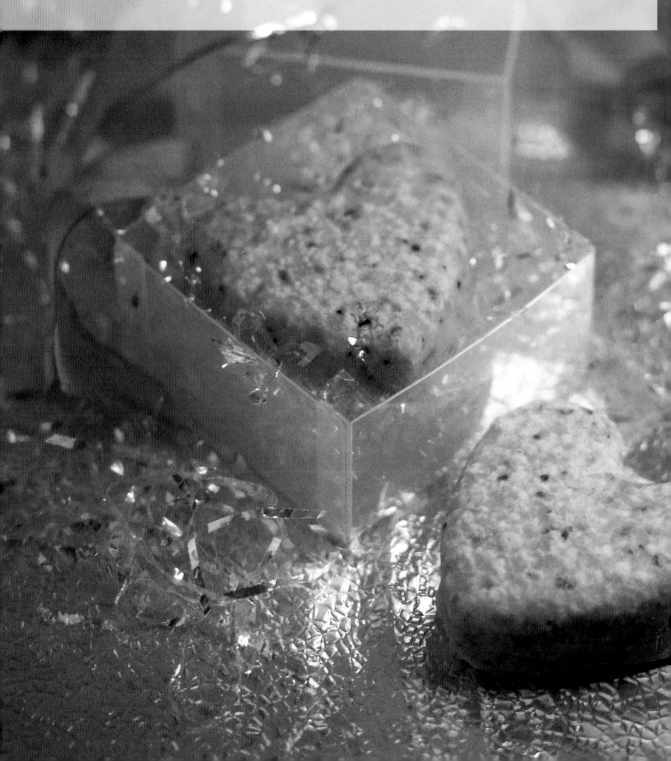

Did You Know? *Dead Sea salts have a well-known reputation for their therapeutic qualities. They are traditionally used in bath and spa products to deeply cleanse and revitalize the skin.*

Moisturizing Bath Bombs

Bath bombs are one of the new additions to bath time products. Their fizz has a really contemporary feel. Yet they are similar to, and based on, the old-fashioned bath tablets that were fashionable a couple of decades ago. Moisturizing bath bombs are different: They don't fizz when they hit the bath water, but sink and then melt, releasing their fragrance and moisturizing oils.

The purpose of moisturizing bath bombs is to provide a richly perfumed, healing softness to the bath water. You can soak, relax, and luxuriate in the silky scented water, while letting the healing qualities of the essential oils, Dead Sea salts, and baking soda soften your skin, and the Monoi de Tahiti moisturize your whole body. Moisturizing bath bombs are a wonderful bath time treat.

Tropical Tang

These bath bombs make a luxuriating bath time treat, and the addition of rosehip granules gives them a delicate, flecked appearance. The fresh smell of bergamot, with just a hint of basil, first arises as the bath bomb melts into the water. Then the calming fragrance of lavender combines with the sensuous aroma of rose to encourage you to lie back and relax.

what's in it?

4 oz (100 gm) baking soda

4 oz (100 gm) Dead Sea salts, finely ground

1 tsp orris root powder

1 heaping tsp laundry starch

½ tsp rosehip granules

3 tbsp Monoi de Tahiti

10 drops rose

10 drops bergamot

10 drops lavender

3 drops basil

how's it made?

1 Place the baking soda, sea salts, orris root powder, and laundry starch in a bowl. Add the rosehip granules and mix thoroughly.

2 Gently warm the Monoi de Tahiti in a double boiler until melted. Add to the dry ingredients, along with the essential oils, and stir well.

3 Spoon or pour the thick, viscous mixture into small, flexible molds. This recipe makes eight bath bombs. Place the molds in the freezer for half an hour.

4 Remove from the molds and leave in a cool, dark place overnight. The bombs will be ready to use in the morning.

Exotic Fizz

Using a base of Monoi de Tahiti gives these moisturizing bath bombs a delicious, exotic perfume. Monoi de Tahiti is a soft, white, waxy substance that comes in a block and melts easily when gently heated. It has the wonderful aroma of gardenia flowers combined with the skin-moisturizing qualities of coconut oil.

what's in it?

4 oz (100 gm) baking soda

4 oz (100 gm) Dead Sea salts, finely ground

1 tsp orris root powder

1 heaping tsp laundry starch

½ tsp finely ground chamomile flowers

3 tbsp Monoi de Tahiti

10 drops rosewood

8 drops chamomile

8 drops lemon

7 drops lime

how's it made?

1 Place the baking soda, sea salts, orris root powder, and laundry starch in a bowl. Add the chamomile flowers and mix thoroughly.

2 Gently warm the Monoi de Tahiti in a double boiler until melted. Add to the dry ingredients, along with the essential oils, and stir well.

3 Spoon or pour the thick, viscous mixture into small, flexible molds. This recipe makes eight bath bombs. Place the molds in the freezer for half an hour.

4 Remove from the molds and leave in a cool, dark place overnight. The bombs will be ready to use in the morning.

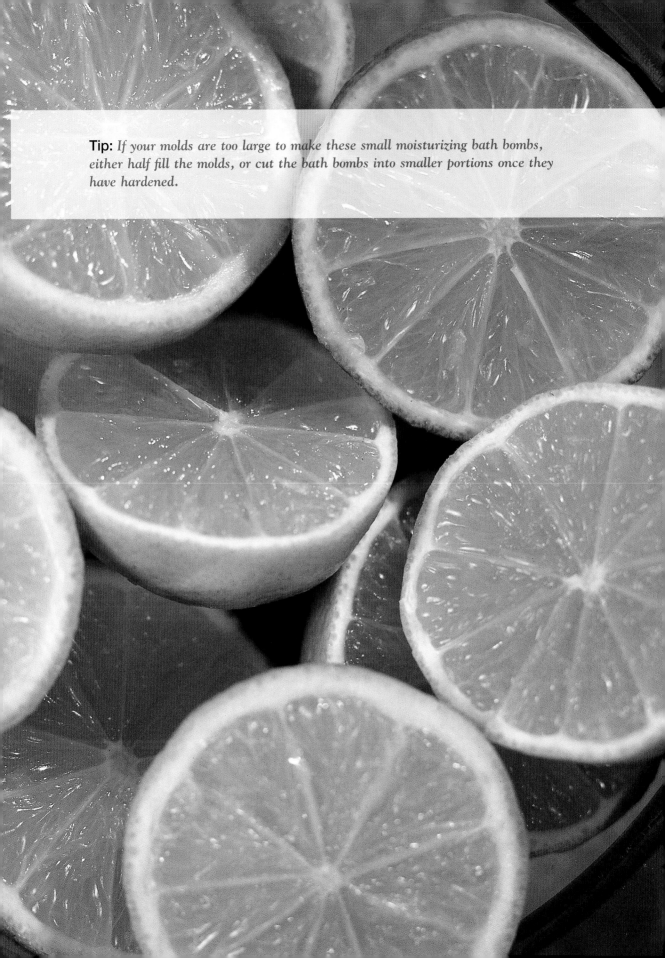

Tip: *If your molds are too large to make these small moisturizing bath bombs, either half fill the molds, or cut the bath bombs into smaller portions once they have hardened.*

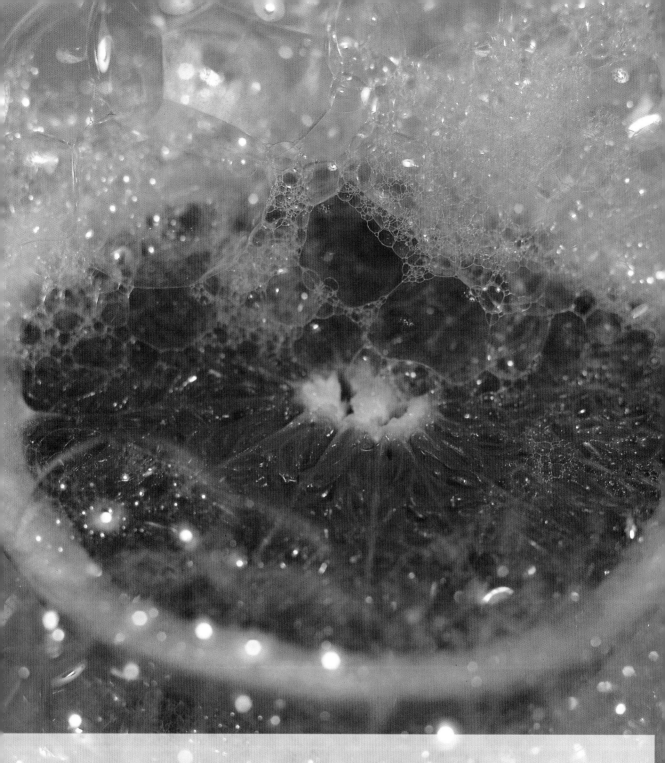

Tip: *To make using Scented Salvation a really relaxing experience, place lighted candles around the bath and turn off the lights. You can play soothing music quietly in the background while you lie back in the warm scented water and let the troubles of the day float away.*

Bubble Baths

Bubble baths are the most familiar of all the bath additives. Their scented, foaming bubbles allow you to lie back and let the soapy water gently float the dirt away. You don't have to scrub yourself down, and you can even do away with using a soap bar altogether if you like.

The popularity of bubble baths means there are many different kinds available. However, the majority of these contain synthetic perfumes and bright chemical colors. These may look good, but they have no real healing qualities and can be harsh on the skin.

Making your own bubble bath is quick and easy, and means you can utilize the healing properties of essential oils and bathe in harmony with nature.

Scented Salvation

We all need rescuing from life's tribulations sometimes, and a bath of Scented Salvation will help you relax. After a long, hard day, the soothing aroma of this bubble bath will float away all your stress and irritability. The sweet, heady fragrance of ylang ylang combines with the clear, calming scent of lavender to help prepare you for sleep. Frankincense helps you breath deeply and let go of stress, while the grapefruit and ginger lift your spirits.

what's in it?
8½ fl oz (250 ml) bubble bath base

9 drops lavender

8 drops ylang ylang

8 drops frankincense

6 drops grapefruit

5 drops ginger

2 drops sandalwood

2 drops jasmine

(Don't worry if you don't have all the essential oils mentioned, as any combination of the above oils will make a delightful, relaxing bath.)

how's it made?

1 Pour the bubble bath base into a container that holds at least 16 fl oz (500 ml) and has a good pouring spout.

2 Carefully drop in the essential oils, one by one, making sure you don't lose count of the drops.

3 Mix the oils thoroughly into the bubble bath base. Be careful not to create too many bubbles. You will see the bubble bath base change slightly. It might seem to turn a little thicker as you stir in the oils, and it will change from clear to opaque.

4 Pour the mixture into a pretty glass bottle (you can use a funnel if you'd like) and the Scented Salvation bubble bath is ready to use.

Winter Warmer

This bubble bath is a powerful ally in the fight against colds, influenza, and all the other coughs, cold, and chills of winter. Incorporating essential oils that help fight off infection, Winter Warmer also includes spice essential oils that warm the mind and body. The familiar smell of eucalyptus combines with the potent aroma of peppermint to provide a powerful antidote to a stuffed-up nose. Lavender soothes sore throats and eases the pain of sinusitis and headaches. Bathing with Winter Warmer can help prevent the onset of a cold as well as relieve its symptoms.

what's in it?

8½ fl oz (250 ml) bubble bath base

9 drops lavender

8 drops eucalyptus

6 drops rosemary

6 drops tea tree

3 drops ginger

4 drops peppermint

2 drops black pepper

(Don't worry if you don't have all the essential oils mentioned, as any combination of the above oils will make a warming bath to help fight off colds and the flu.)

how's it made?

1 Pour the bubble bath base into a container that holds at least 16 fl oz (500 ml) and has a good pouring spout.

2 Carefully drop in the essential oils, one by one, making sure you don't lose count of the drops.

3 Mix the oils thoroughly into the bubble bath base. Be careful not to create too many bubbles. You will see the bubble bath base change slightly. It might seem to turn a little thicker as you stir in the oils, and it will change from clear to opaque.

4 Pour the mixture into a pretty glass bottle (you can use a funnel if you'd like) and the Winter Warmer bubble bath is now ready to use.

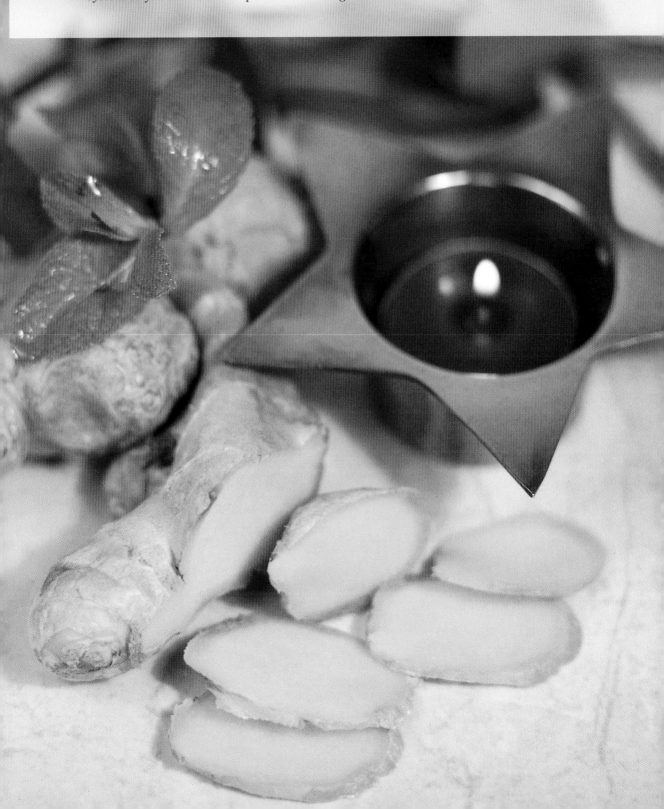

Did You Know? *Tea tree is one of nature's most powerful anti-infectious agents, successfully warding off viruses as well as bacteria and fungi. Tea tree is also an immuno-stimulant. This means it helps the body strengthen its immune system so you are less susceptible to catching viruses.*

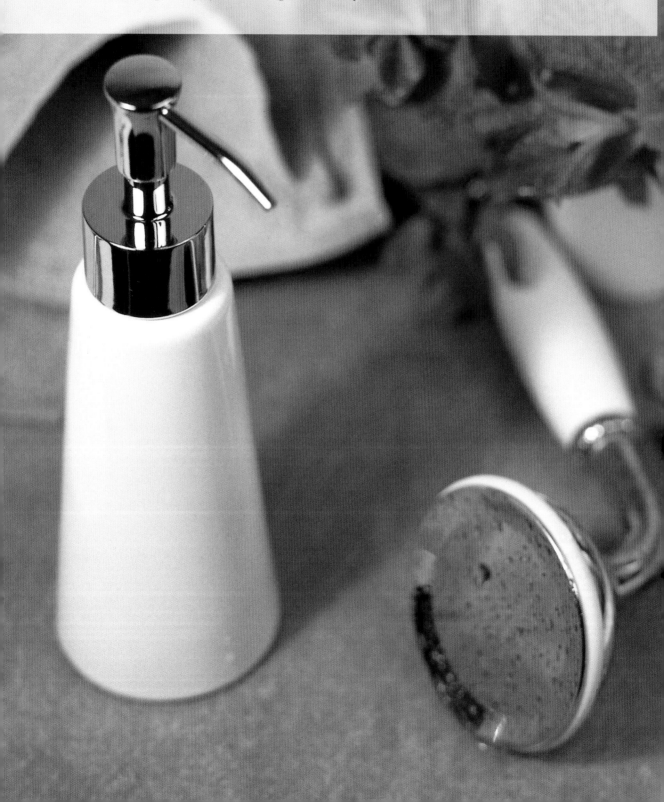

Did You Know? *Peppermint contains a lot of menthol—an excellent decongestant—so Minty Spice is a good shower gel to use when you have a cold. Peppermint also has a mildly antiseptic effect, which helps deeply cleanse the skin, especially after sweating out the body's toxins.*

Shower Gels

Shower gels are a better alternative to soap bars in the shower. Even while using a draining soap dish, most bars of soap—especially natural, organic vegetable soaps, which tend to be softer than commercially made soaps—will disintegrate quickly and be wasted. Shower gels are equally, if not more, effective than bars of soap and they won't melt away on their own. The addition of essential oils to the shower gel base creates a fresh smelling, pleasant-to-use body wash.

To some extent, shower gel and bubble bath bases are similar, though bubble bath is often made from a thicker base product. The thickness of shower gel and bubble bath depends on which supplier you purchase your base products from. This means shower gel and bubble bath bases can be interchanged, according to personal preference. It is best to try out both your base products in the bath and the shower, and decide which you like best in each circumstance.

Minty Spice

This recipe is very freshening and deodorant, so it makes a good shower gel to use after lounging in a sauna, playing sports, or participating in other strenuous activities. The addition of peppermint essential oil gives you a light, tingly feeling all over, while the clean, clear smell of the citrus and spice oils refresh your senses. Minty Spice leaves your skin feeling toned and clean.

what's in it?

8½ fl oz (250 ml) shower gel base
10 drops green color (see page 126)
10 drops palmarosa
10 drops peppermint
8 drops coriander
6 drops lemon
4 drops bergamot
2 drops clove

how's it made?

1 Pour the shower gel base into a container that holds at least 16 fl oz (500 ml) and has a good pouring spout. Add the green color.

2 Carefully drop in all the essential oils, one by one.

3 Mix the oils thoroughly into the shower gel base. Be careful not to create too many bubbles. The mixture will turn from clear to opaque as you mix in the essential oils.

4 Pour the mixture into a squeeze bottle, or pump-dispenser bottle, and the Minty Spice shower gel is ready to use.

Early Riser

Waking up isn't always that easy, especially after a late night. Early Riser contains essential oils that are fresh smelling and stimulating to wake you up and help you face the day ahead. This shower gel is best used only in the morning, as the stimulating oils are counter-productive for sleep. Even after the heaviest night out, you will feel refreshed and ready to go after a shower with Early Riser.

what's in it?

8½ fl oz (250 ml) shower gel base

10 drops geranium

10 drops bergamot

8 drops rosemary

6 drops petitgrain

4 drops juniper

2 drops basil

how's it made?

1 Pour the shower gel base into a container that holds at least 16 fl oz (500 ml) and has a good pouring spout.

2 Carefully drop in all the essential oils, one by one.

3 Mix the oils thoroughly into the shower gel base. Be careful not to create too many bubbles. The mixture will turn from clear to opaque as you mix in the essential oils.

4 Pour the mixture into a squeeze bottle, or pump-dispenser bottle, and the Early Riser shower gel is ready to use.

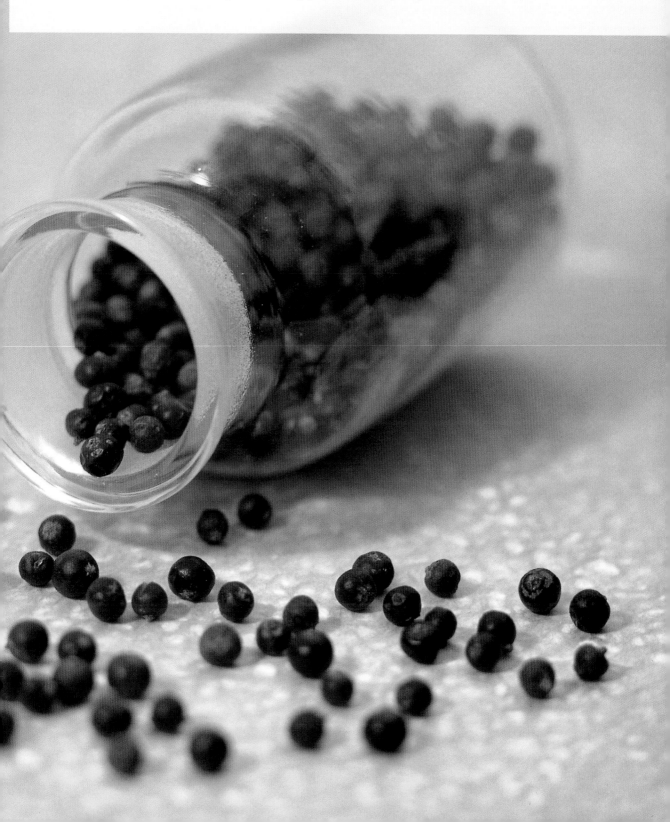

Tip: *Plastic squeeze bottles are the traditional containers for shower gels, and they work quite well. However, using a pump-action dispenser bottle is even easier, so that when your hands are slippery with suds you don't have to hold and squeeze the bottle; you need only press the pump dispenser.*

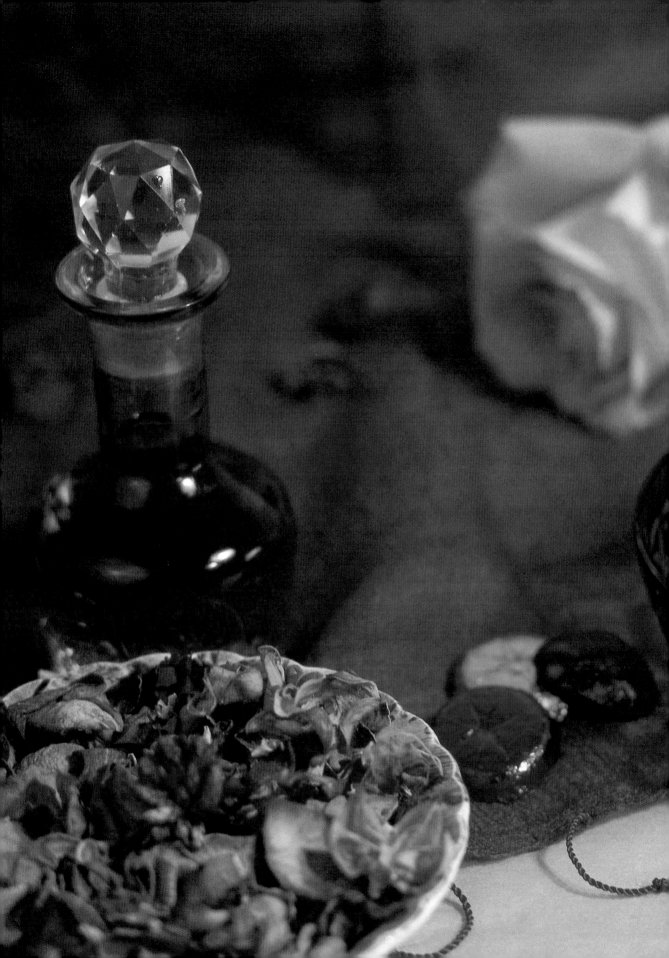

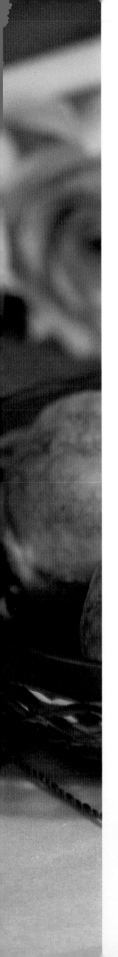

Chapter 11

Cream Soaps, Hand-Milled Soaps, and Wash Balls

Handcrafted Soaps

In this chapter you will learn how to make a range of simple, handcrafted soaps. The techniques involved in making these soaps are a little more sophisticated than the techniques for making the recipes from the previous chapter, but not quite as demanding as making the cold-process soaps in the next chapter. Cream soaps, hand-milled soaps, and wash balls all provide the opportunity to make your own soaps simply and quickly, yet the finished product can look wonderful and professional if you spend some time and imagination in wrapping and presenting the soaps in creative ways.

Cream soaps are made by using ready-bought soap flakes as the main ingredient. Some soap flakes are derived from professionally produced machine-milled soap that has been grated into fine flakes. Professionally milled soap is made by machines that press freshly made soap between rollers. This process flattens the bar into a very thin sheet, which is then shredded into soap flakes. This flattening and shredding is repeated several times. The mixture is then put through an extruding machine that condenses the mixture into bars of tightly compacted soap so that the individual flakes are no longer discernible.

These bars of soap are what you typically purchase in the drugstore or supermarket. The bars of soap are very hard and have a polished appearance, and the milling process has given the soaps a quick and easy lathering quality. These bars of soap can withstand being dropped in the bath or basin without disintegrating. However, the majority of machine-milled soaps are made from beef tallow and various synthetic additives. This means that they are not of pure vegetable origin nor are they organic—a good reason to ensure that you buy only natural, vegetable-based soap flakes.

Making your own hand-milled soap is both simple and creative. Start by purchasing some bars of unscented, uncolored vegetable soap. Using a kitchen grater, grate the bars to produce fine curls of soap that are easy to melt down. Making hand-milled soap is also a great way to use up any leftover pieces of quality soap that have become too small to use.

The wash balls recipes in this book are derived and adapted from one of the early, more traditional forms of soap. Before commercially produced soap became available, wash balls were traditionally used in both the kitchen and bathroom, for all washing and laundry purposes. The coarsest and most basic wash balls would be used to launder clothes and linens, while the more elaborate soap balls—often perfumed with flowers, flower waters, and herbs—would be used for personal washing.

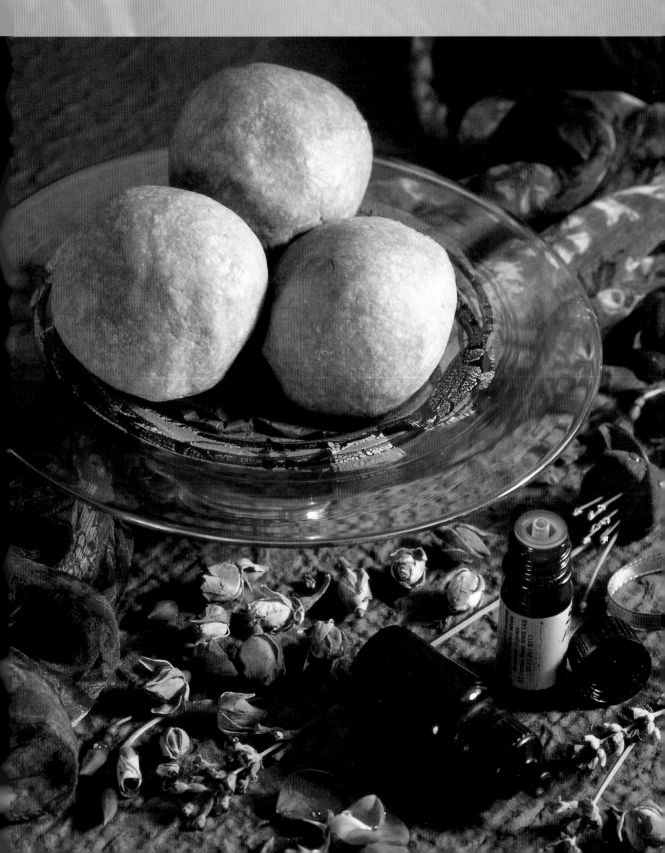

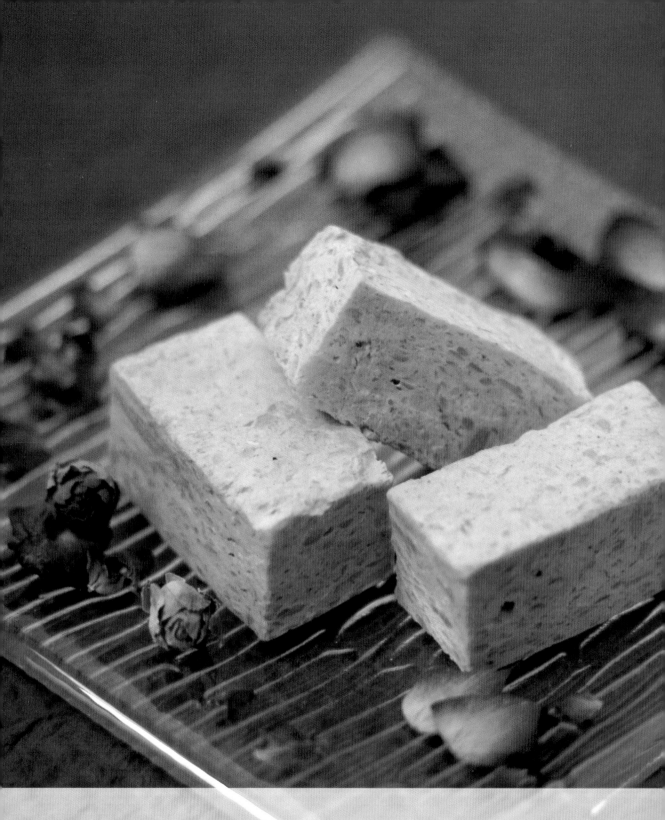

Tip: *To make a romantic present for a loved one you could place the Honey Rose Dream soap in a pretty box on a bed of dried rose petals.*

Cream Soaps

Cream soap recipes are created using soap flakes. You can purchase soap flakes from any of the specialty suppliers on pages 222–223, but they are also available from good quality drugstores. You do need to check that the soap flakes you purchase are made purely from soap with no detergent, color, or perfume added.

The soap flakes are slowly melted with liquid glycerin (and sometimes a base oil, such as almond oil) over a double boiler. The addition of a base oil makes a lighter weight soap. Once all the flakes have melted, the mixture is removed from the heat and essential oils, natural colors, and any other ingredients are added. Finally, the mixture is whipped either with a hand whisk or an electric beater. This makes the soap light and creamy, but it thickens in just a few minutes. As soon as the mixture has thickened, spoon the cream soap into a greased mold and leave it to set in a cool place.

Honey Rose Dream

The healing qualities of honey are incorporated in this mild soap, which makes the soap soft and sweet. The addition of rosehip granules gives the soap a delicate pinky-peach color and the voluptuous scent of roses makes it smell like a dream.

what's in it?

8 oz (225 gm) soap flakes
6¾ fl oz (200 ml) rose water
1 tbsp (15 ml) honey
1 tbsp (15 ml) almond oil
1 tbsp (10 ml) liquid glycerin
1 large tsp rosehip granules
25 drops rose
10 drops neroli
10 drops chamomile
5 drops frankincense

how's it made?

1 Place the soap flakes, rosewater, honey, almond oil, and glycerin over a double boiler and heat until the soap flakes melt. Stir with a glass stirring rod or chopstick to blend the mixture thoroughly.

2 Add the rosehip granules and stir. The mixture will turn a pinky-peach color.

3 Remove from the heat and carefully drop in the essential oils, one by one, and then whisk the mixture with an electric beater until it thickens, in a few minutes.

4 Quickly spoon the mixture into a greased mold, and smooth off with the back of a spoon dipped in hot water.

5 Let set for an hour, or until the soap is firm to the touch, and then turn it out of the mold.

6 Leave to dry on waxed paper for two to three weeks. The Honey Rose Dream cream soap will then be ready to use.

Indian Promise

This soap is left uncolored so you end up with a pale, creamy, natural-looking soap. The exotic scent is reminiscent of the Orient, with its warm, spicy fragrance. The addition of jojoba oil makes a light soap with excellent moisturizing qualities, so this is a good soap to use if you have dry skin.

what's in it?

8 oz (225 gm) soap flakes
6¾ fl oz (200 ml) orange flower water
2 tbsp (25 ml) jojoba oil
1 tbsp (10 ml) liquid glycerin
1 tbsp (5 ml) cocoa butter
20 drops sandalwood
10 drops ginger
5 drops coriander
5 drops cinnamon
5 drops lemongrass
5 drops vanilla

how's it made?

1 Place the soap flakes, orange flower water, jojoba oil, and glycerin over a double boiler. Heat gently until the soap flakes start to melt. Stir with a glass stirring rod or chopstick to blend the mixture thoroughly.

2 Melt the cocoa butter in a small saucepan, and add to the melted ingredients.

3 Remove from the heat and carefully drop in the essential oils, one by one, and then whisk the mixture with an electric beater until it thickens, in a few minutes.

4 Quickly spoon the mixture into a greased mold, and smooth off with the back of a spoon dipped in hot water.

5 Let set for an hour, or until the soap is firm to the touch, and then turn it out of the mold.

6 Leave to dry on waxed paper for two to three weeks the Indian Promise cream soap will then be ready to use.

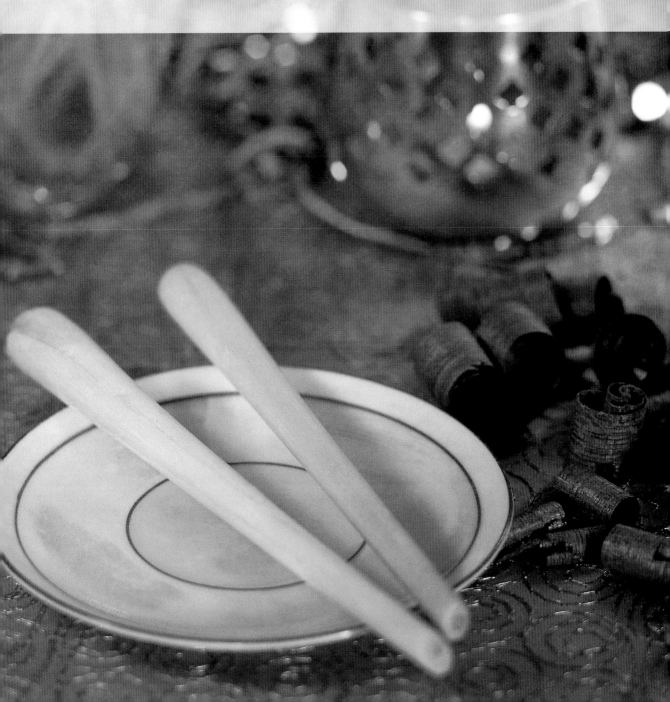

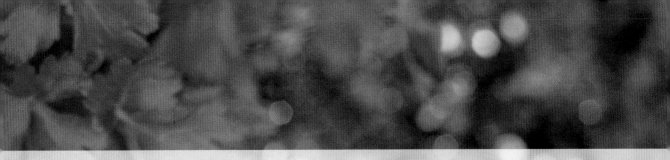

Did You Know? *Traditionally, spices (and thus their scents) are used to stimulate the appetite. Many of the essential oils used in Indian Promise are also used in Indian and other Asian cooking. Sandalwood has been used in India for centuries in Ayurvedic skin care preparations and to perfume soap.*

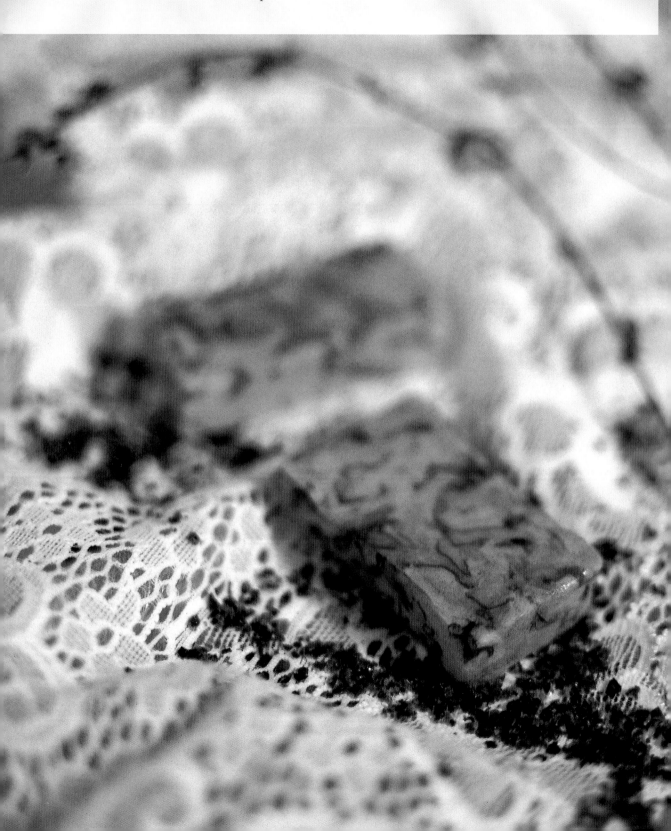

Tip: *The addition of rose petals gives a marbled, textured effect to the Summer Seduction hand-milled soap.*

Hand-Milled Soaps

In addition to grating bars of soap and recycling leftover soap pieces, you can also use the trimmings from your soap making efforts to make hand-milled soap. It doesn't take long to accumulate enough leftovers and trimmings to make a batch of hand-milled soap. However, when you use leftover soap scraps and trimmings, remember to add less essential oils and colors, as these scraps of soap are already colored and perfumed.

Homemade hand-milled soap produces a softer, fluffier, and less durable soap. However, making and using your own natural soap is more pleasurable than using the longer-lasting, synthetic, store-bought variety. These recipes include various additions to make colored, textured, and fragrant soaps. Once you have made a few batches of soap, you can then experiment with different ingredients. In this way, you can create your own personalized hand-milled soaps.

Summer Seduction

This sweet smelling soap has a romantic pinky-peach color because of the addition of rosehip granules. Shea butter is also known as African karite butter. It soothes and softens dry or chapped skin and nourishes all skin types. The inclusion of shea butter makes a gentle soap that is suitable for people with sensitive skin.

what's in it?

18 fl oz (530 ml) water

1 tbsp (10 gm) rosehip granules

8 oz (225 gm) grated, unscented, uncolored, vegetable-based soap

1 oz (30 ml) beeswax

1 oz (30 ml) shea butter

1 tsp (5 gm) rose petals or dried rosebuds (optional)

20 drops rosewood

10 drops rose

10 drops bergamot

10 drops patchouli

5 drops ylang ylang

5 drops vetiver

how's it made?

1 Grease enough molds for approximatley twelve bars of soap with a little sunflower oil. Put the water in the top half of a double boiler. If you don't have a double boiler, you can fit a small saucepan inside a bigger one. Add the rosehip granules and grated soap slowly, stirring gently as you mix the soap into the water.

2 Either let the soap melt thoroughly, stirring frequently, or alternatively, pour into a blender and blend until the mixture is smooth. You may need to add a little more water.

3 When the soap is fully melted, add the beeswax and shea butter. Stir until melted. If you blended the soap and water, pour back into the pan and stir gently to remove as much air as possible. Then add the beeswax and shea butter.

4 Remove from the heat and gently stir in the rose petals, if using. Finally, add the essential oils and incorporate them into the mixture.

5 Pour the soap into the greased molds, and cover with plastic wrap. After twenty-four hours, remove the plastic wrap and place molds in a warm, dry place for another twenty-four hours. Then take the soap bars out of the molds and place on waxed paper.

6 If you used one large mold, after a week, trim the top, bottom, and edges of the block of soap and cut into individual bars. Check the soap bars are drying out and hardening nicely every ten days or so, and flip them. Trim off any discolored or uneven edges. The soap will be ready in about three weeks.

Oatmeal and Honey

*This is a gently exfoliating, soothing soap, and
an enduring, traditional favorite. Oatmeal adds
texture to the lather and helps you gently scrub
away dead skin cells. Honey hydrates, soothes,
and moisturizes the skin. Cocoa butter is rich,
soothing, and softening.*

what's in it?

18 fl oz (530 ml) water

8 oz (225 gm) grated, unscented, uncolored, vegetable-
    based soap

1 oz (30 ml) beeswax

1 oz (30 ml) cocoa butter

1 tbsp (15 gm) finely ground oatmeal

1 tbsp (15 ml) gently warmed honey

5 drops vanilla

20 drops nutmeg

20 drops sandalwood

15 drops orange

how's it made?

1 Grease enough molds for approximately twelve
bars of soap with a little sunflower oil. Put the
water in the top half of a double boiler, and heat
until nearly boiling. If you don't have a double
boiler, you can fit a small saucepan inside a bigger
one. Add the grated soap slowly, stirring gently as
you mix the soap into the water.

2 Grated soap can take an hour or so to melt
thoroughly and requires frequent stirring.
Alternatively, you can stir the mixture for five
minutes until you have a glutinous mixture and
the grated soap curls are beginning to disintegrate. Then pour into a blender and blend until
the mixture is smooth. You may need to add a little more water.

3 When the soap is fully melted, add the
beeswax and cocoa butter. Stir until melted.
If you blended the soap and water, pour back into
the pan and stir gently to remove as much air as
possible. Then add the beeswax and cocoa butter.

4 Remove from the heat and pour in the oatmeal, stirring to mix it in thoroughly. Finally
add the honey and essential oils and incorporate
them into the mixture.

5 Pour the soap into the greased molds and
cover with plastic wrap. After twenty-four
hours, remove the plastic wrap and place molds in
a warm, dry place for another twenty-four hours.
Then take the soap bars out of the molds and place
on waxed paper.

6 If you used one large mold, after a week, trim
the top, bottom, and edges of the block of soap
and cut into individual bars. Check the soap bars
are drying out and hardening nicely every ten days
or so, and flip them. Trim off any discolored or
uneven edges. The soap will be ready in about
three weeks.

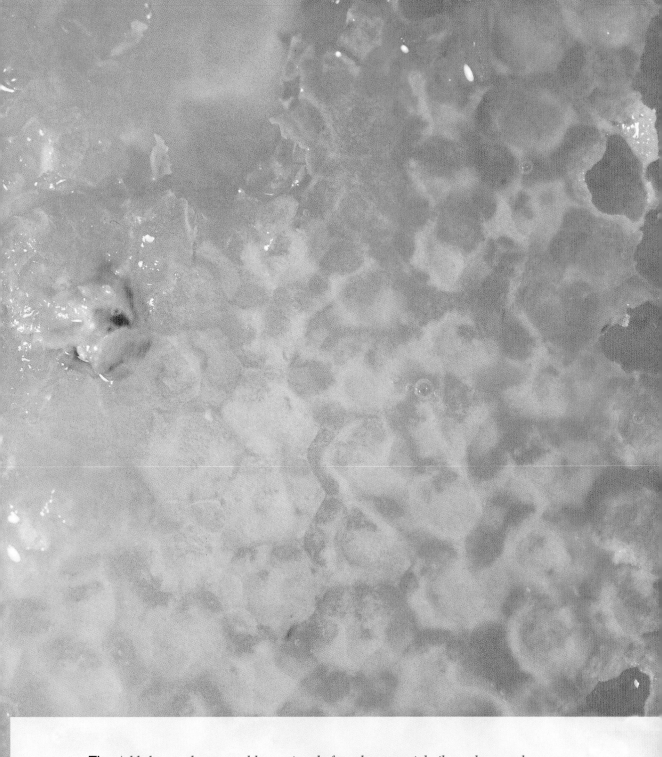

Tip: *Add the gently warmed honey just before the essential oils so the soap has cooled slightly. High temperatures destroy the honey's active properties.*

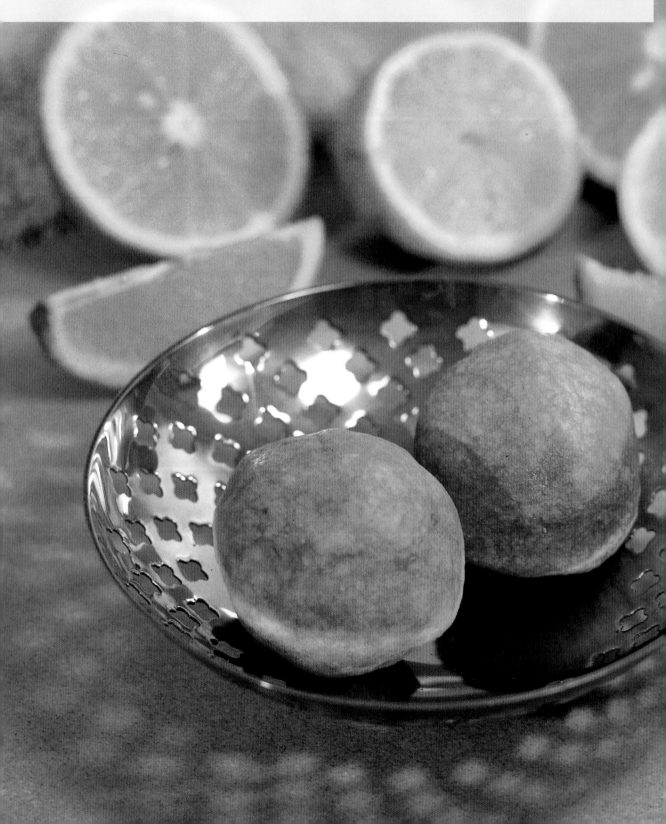

Did You Know? *Halved lemons were traditionally kept near the kitchen sink and used to rub over the hands to dispel the powerful aroma of onions and garlic. This citrus soap makes a good alternative and is pleasant to use in the kitchen.*

Wash Balls

Wash balls are yet another example of how you can make homemade soap in your kitchen. The recipes below are specially designed to make easily molded wash balls, and the ingredients include binding agents such as laundry starch and orris root powder. Orris root is primarily used in the perfume industry as a fixative, which means that orris root literally anchors the scent into an overall fragrance. When it is used to make wash balls, it both acts as a fixative and as a binding agent.

You can also make soap balls from cold-process soap to achieve a different effect. After about a week during cold-process curing, the soap is firm enough to handle yet soft enough to still be malleable. Simply scoop up a handful of soap and roll into a ball (be sure to wear rubber gloves). To make snow balls, make sure the soap is still quite moist. After shaping it into a ball, roll it in finely shaved white soap. To achieve a different effect, roll it in finely ground flower petals or oatmeal.

Orange Lemon Tang

This sharp and sweet smelling soap contains a combination of citrus essential oils and other lemon- and orange-scented oils. This makes a clean, refreshing perfumed soap with just a hint of floral sweetness.

what's in it?

8 oz (225 gm) soap flakes
1 tsp (5 ml) orris root powder
1 tsp (5 ml) laundry starch
15 drops orange
15 drops lemon
10 drops mandarin
10 drops petitgrain
5 drops lemongrass
5 drops bergamot
5 drops rosewood
5 drops geranium
1 tbsp (15 ml) almond oil
1 tbsp (10 ml) orange or yellow color, according to
 preference (see page 126)
5 tbsp (75 ml) hot orange flower water

how's it made?

1 Grind the soap flakes with a pestle and mortar until you have a fine, gritty powder. Pour into a mixing bowl.

2 Add the orris root powder and laundry starch and mix well. Add the essential oils to the almond oil, then add to the dry ingredients, along with the color of your choice, and mix well.

3 Add the hot orange flower water to the bowl and mix everything together well with a fork.

4 As the mixture starts to bind, use your hands to knead it until you achieve a uniform, pliable dough. Divide the mixture into three roughly equal-sized pieces and roll into balls.

5 Grease your hands lightly with sunflower oil and continue to mold the balls until all irregularities are smoothed out.

6 Place on waxed paper in a warm, dry space for five days. The Orange Lemon Tang wash balls will then be ready to use.

Chocolate Spice

Using real, organic chocolate makes these wash balls smell delicious, and almost good enough to eat. The chocolate and the ground cinnamon give the soap a lovely, rich, earthy brown color. If you have children around, make sure they know these Chocolate Spice wash balls are soap and are not edible!

what's in them?

8 oz (225 gm) soap flakes

1 tbsp (15 ml) organic cocoa or dark chocolate powder

1 tsp (5 ml) laundry starch

2 tbsp (25 ml) apricot kernel oil

½ tsp (2.5 ml) ground cinnamon

10 drops nutmeg

10 drops cinnamon

5 drops cardamon

5 drops vanilla

5 tbsp (75 ml) hot water

how're they made?

1 Grind the soap flakes with a pestle and mortar until you have a fine, gritty powder. Pour into a mixing bowl.

2 Add the cocoa powder and laundry starch and mix well. Add the essential oils to the apricot kernel oil, add to the dry ingredients, and mix well.

3 Add the hot water to the bowl and mix everything together well with a fork.

4 As the mixture starts to bind, use your hands to knead it until you achieve a uniform, pliable dough. Divide the mixture into three roughly equal-sized pieces and roll into balls.

5 Grease your hands lightly with sunflower oil and continue to mold the balls until all irregularities are smoothed out.

6 Place on waxed paper in a warm, dry space for five days. The Chocolate Spice wash balls will then be ready to use.

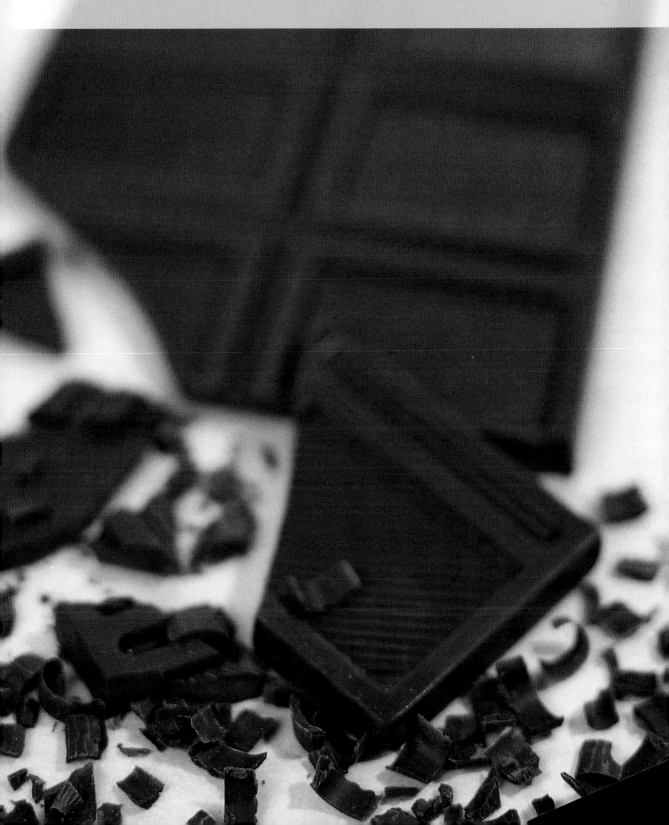

Tip: *Washing or bathing with milk was a traditional way of keeping the skin soft. Most famously, Cleopatra bathed in asses' milk. To make a creamy milk chocolate soap, substitute goat's milk, cow's milk, or oat milk for the water.*

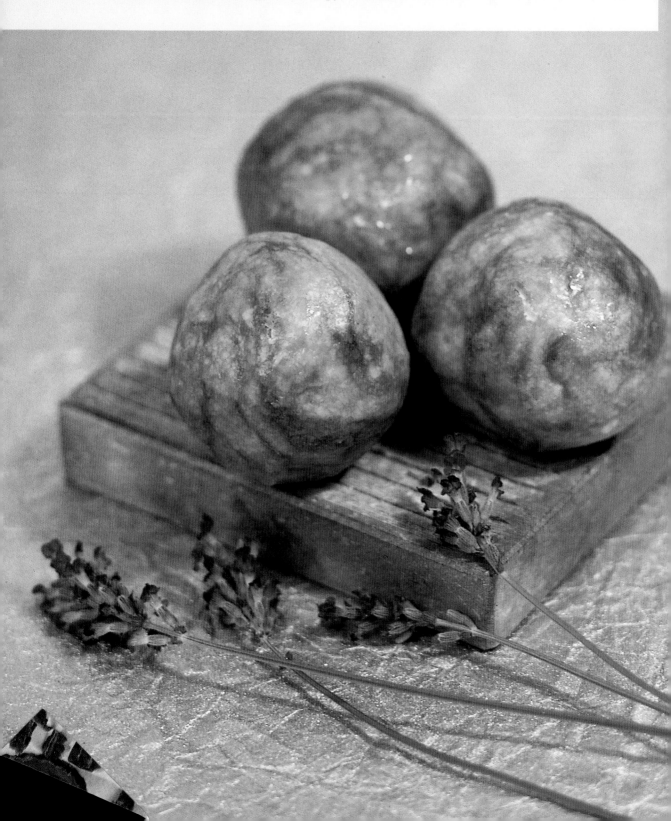

Tip: When you mix in the red color with your fingers, be prepared for pinky-red stains on your fingertips from the strong color base. This will fade in a day or two, or can be scrubbed off with a soapy nail brush.

Purple Marble

These dramatic looking wash balls have lovely alternating swirls of purple and peachy pink. The marbled effect is created by mixing in the color at the end, after the soap is made. The scent is rich and deep, with resinous and woody undertones, together with light, fresh, and sweet floral top notes.

what's in it?

8 oz (225 gm) soap flakes
1 tsp (5 ml) orris root powder
1 tsp (5 ml) laundry starch
1 tbsp (10 ml) shea butter, melted
15 drops frankincense
15 drops sandalwood
10 drops patchouli
10 drops geranium
10 drops bergamot
5 drops rose
5 drops ylang ylang
5 tbsp (75 ml) hot rose water
2 tbsp (25 ml) red color (see page 126)

how's it made?

1 Grind the soap flakes with a pestle and mortar until you have a fine, gritty powder. Pour into a mixing bowl.

2 Add the orris root powder and laundry starch and mix well. Add the essential oils to the dry ingredients, along with the hot melted shea butter, and mix well.

3 Pour the hot rose water into the bowl and mix everything together well with a fork.

4 As the mixture starts to bind, use your hands to knead it until you achieve a uniform, pliable dough. Add the red color and blend into the dough with your fingertips to create a marbled effect. Divide the mixture into three roughly equal-sized pieces and roll into balls.

5 Grease your hands lightly with sunflower oil and continue to mold the balls until all irregularities are smoothed out.

6 Place on waxed paper in a warm, dry space for five days. The Purple Marble wash balls will then be ready to use.

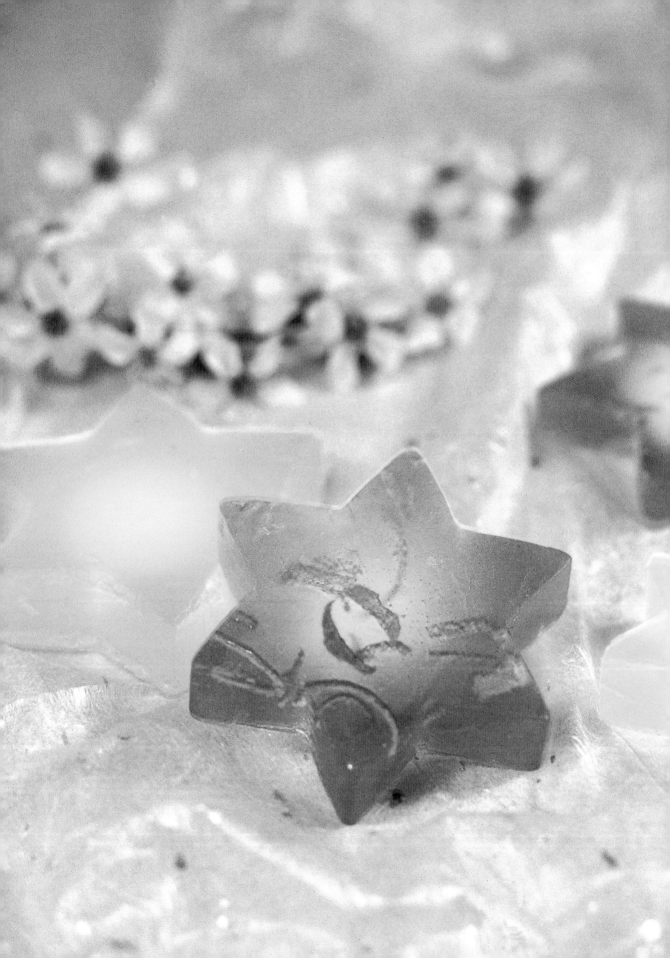

Chapter 12

Glycerin Soaps and Cold-Process Vegetable Soaps

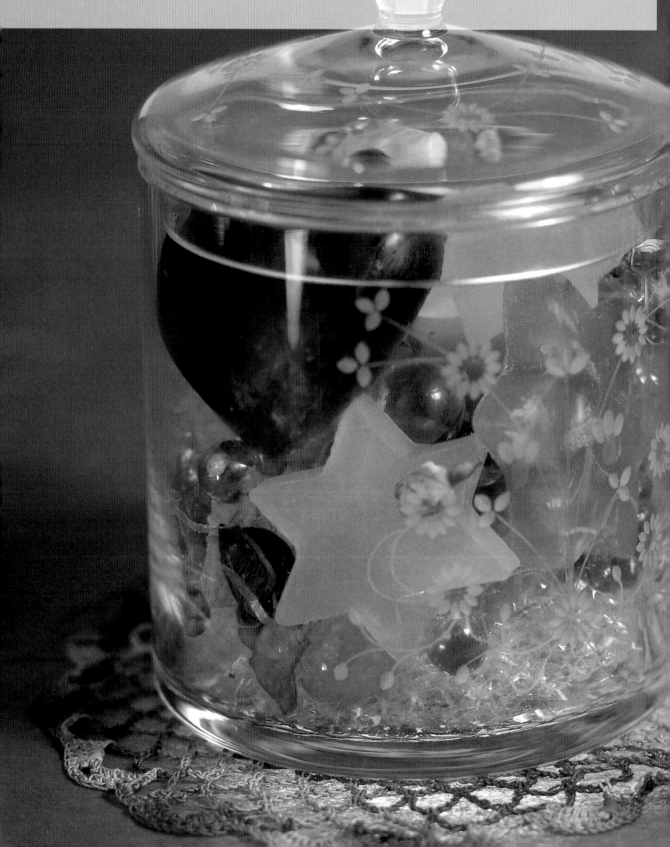

Making Real Soap

The cold-process vegetable soaps in this chapter are the most complicated to make. They take time and effort, and you might need to practice a few batches to get the hang of the process. Nonetheless, making your own natural soap from scratch is a really rewarding activity. Once you have made and used a successful batch of hand-crafted soap, you may find you never again want to buy commercially produced soap.

As the quotation on page 168 suggests, it is helpful for the newcomer to soap making to learn as much as possible at first. One of the most important ideas to keep in mind is how to choose your basic ingredients. This book advocates the organic, natural philosophy, and uses organic and vegetable-based ingredients. Ingredients for commercially made soap are usually selected for cheapness and the physical properties they will bring to the finished soap. However, you can choose organic base ingredients that first and foremost have good skin-care properties. It is a good idea to read about the different skin-care qualities of the wide range of base oils and nutrients now available.

The quotation also encourages you to be creative once you've learned the basic techniques of making soap. Soap making can be an art form if you invest the process with the vision, creative impulse, and passion of the artist. Beautiful soaps, presented in unusual and attractive packaging, can adorn a bathroom—alongside being useful, of course!

They also make wonderful gifts, and there are ideas on how to display, wrap, and present your soaps in chapter fourteen (see pages 206–215).

Don't worry if some batches of cold-process soap don't work out. The most important thing is to figure out and understand why something went wrong. In this way, you can try not to repeat the mistake again. However, making soap involves a little magic and luck, and even the most experienced soap maker can end up with a batch of soap that's not quite right, or even a complete flop. There is a section on troubleshooting at the end of the book that explains why common problems happen and how to avoid them (see page 218).

Making the glycerin soaps is much simpler and quicker, and provides a good contrast to the time and effort involved in making cold-process soap. You could probably start a batch of cold-process soap and during the time it takes to cure and finish, you could have made and used up a bar of glycerin soap! Yet these two different kinds of soap do have something in common that distinguishes them from the previous recipes. Both cold-process and glycerin soaps are made and sold commercially, while all the other soaps are handcrafted specialties that you would be unlikely to find for sale in your local drugstore. So, if soap making really inspires you, perhaps one day you may swell the numbers of cottage industry soap makers.

Glycerin Soaps

Glycerin soaps are increasingly fashionable these days. The first soap ever to be widely advertised was Pears Soap, which is a glycerin soap with a floral and herbal fragrance. Pears fell from favor with the introduction of commercially produced, machine-milled soap. A huge range of these soaps was created and dominated the market. However, with the renewed interest in glycerin soaps, Pears Soap is now proving popular once again.

The process of making glycerin soap is simple: melt a block glycerin, add color and perfume, and allow it to set for an hour or two. This means making these soaps is almost instantly gratifying, and is definitely fun, rather than hard, work. As most of these soaps are nearly transparent, you can add little treasures that are slowly exposed through washing. Little plastic animals, marbles, crystals, and other small ornaments all make decorative and fun additions.

Sweet Hearts

Intriguing and beautiful, these soaps are created by using a flexible, heart-shaped mold, though you can use different shaped molds for other looks if you prefer. These striking soaps are infused with the delicate scent of roses, and the soft, fresh aroma of bergamot. The intense, opaque shade of purple comes from using a lot of red base color.

what's in it?

8 oz (225 gm) grated block glycerin
20 drops red color (see page 126)
20 drops rose
15 drops neroli
15 drops bergamot

how's it made?

1 Grease a heart-shaped mold with a little sunflower oil. Put the grated block glycerin in the top half of a double boiler, or use two saucepans as described on page 157, and heat until melted, stirring gently with a chopstick or glass stirring rod.

2 Remove from the heat and gently stir in the red color, followed by the essential oils. The mixture will turn an intense purple color.

3 Pour the soap into the greased mold. Leave to set for about one and a half hours, or until firm to the touch.

4 Once the soap is set, turn out of the mold. The Sweet Hearts glycerin soap is now ready to use.

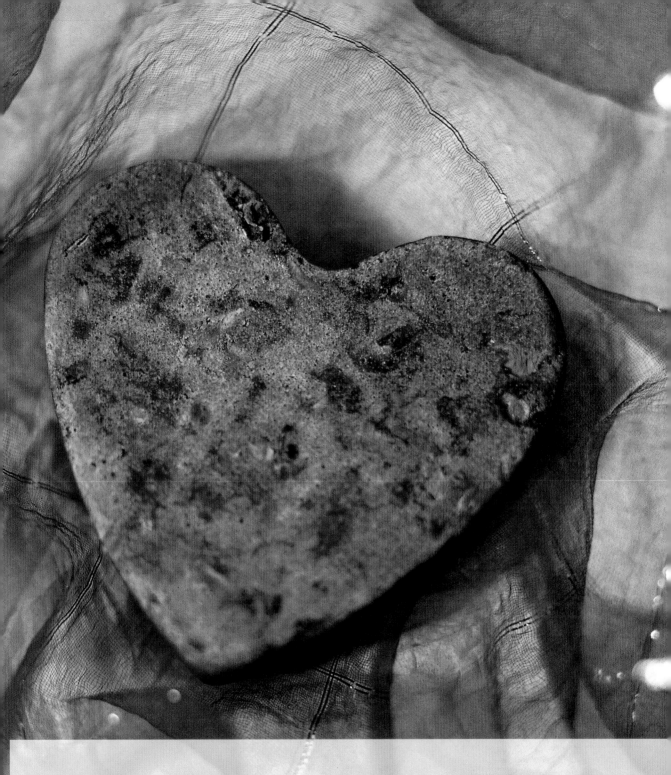

Tip: *For extra effect, you can press a single dried rosebud into the surface of the soap just after pouring it into the mold.*

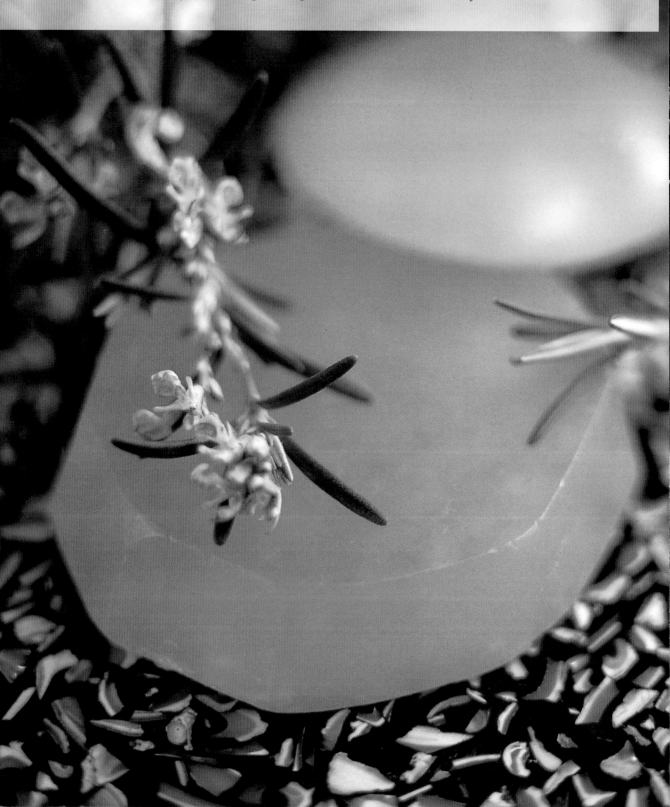

Did You Know? *Many of the herbal essential oils and lavender were used as traditional strewing herbs in the Middle Ages. They were mixed in with rushes and used as floor coverings to keep bad smells and insects away.*

Herbal Garden

The fresh, green aroma of this soap is evocative of a traditional herb garden on a hot summer's day. The addition of blue chamomile gives the soap a delicate, natural blue-green color, as do some types of vetivert. Lavender adds a delicate floral note.

what's in it?

8 oz (225 gm) grated block glycerin
10 drops lavender
5 drops rosemary
5 drops basil
5 drops sweet marjoram
15 drops blue chamomile
10 drops vetivert

how's it made?

1 Grease a mold with a little sunflower oil. Put the grated block glycerin in the top half of a double boiler, or use two saucepans as described on page 157, and heat until melted, stirring gently with a chopstick or glass stirring rod.

2 Remove from the heat and gently stir in the essential oils. The mixture will turn a delicate blue-green color.

3 Pour the soap into the greased mold. Leave to set for about one and a half hours, or until firm to the touch.

4 Once the soap is set, turn out of the mold and trim into whatever shape you like. The Herbal Garden glycerin soap is now ready to use.

Sweet and Spicy

This lovely, fragrant soap will appeal to both women and men. Sweet and Spicy is a good soap to use in the morning, as it has an invigorating, uplifting aroma. The ground cinnamon gives the soap a speckled brown appearance, while the addition of spice essential oils means the soap has a slightly warming effect on the skin.

what's in it?

8 oz (225 gm) grated block glycerin
10 drops ginger
5 drops cardamon
5 drops clove
10 drops cinnamon
10 drops grapefruit
5 drops ylang ylang
5 drops geranium
1 tsp (5 ml) finely ground cinnamon

how's it made?

1 Grease a mold with a little sunflower oil. Put the grated block glycerin in the top half of a double boiler, or use two saucepans as described on page 157, and heat until melted, stirring gently with a chopstick or glass stirring rod.

2 Remove from the heat and gently stir in the essential oils and the ground cinnamon. The mixture will turn a warm, brown color.

3 Pour the soap into the greased mold. Leave to set for about one and a half hours, or until firm to the touch.

4 Once the soap is set, turn out of the mold and trim into whatever shape you like. The Sweet and Spicy glycerin soap is now ready to use.

Marmalade Star

Using a star-shaped cookie cutter makes this a really fun soap to make and wash with. Children especially love using Marmalade Star and they also like helping to make it. The vibrant orange color and the sweet, warm scent of orange combined with slivers of orange peel make this soap reminiscent of marmalade.

what's in it?

8 oz (225 gm) grated block glycerin

50 drops orange

5 drops orange color (see page 126)

1 tsp (5 ml) finely sliced orange peel without the pith

how's it made?

1 Grease a rectangular mold with a little sun-flower oil. Put the grated block glycerin in the top half of a double boiler, or use two saucepans as described on page 157, and heat until melted, stirring gently with a chopstick or glass stirring rod.

2 Remove from the heat and gently stir in the essential oil, the orange color, and the slivers of orange peel. The mixture will turn a bright orange color.

3 Pour the soap into the greased mold. Leave to set for about one and a half hours, or until firm to the touch.

4 Once the soap is set, turn out of the mold. Using a star shaped cookie cutter, press firmly down on the soap to cut out two Marmalade Star glycerin soaps. The Marmalade Star is now ready to use.

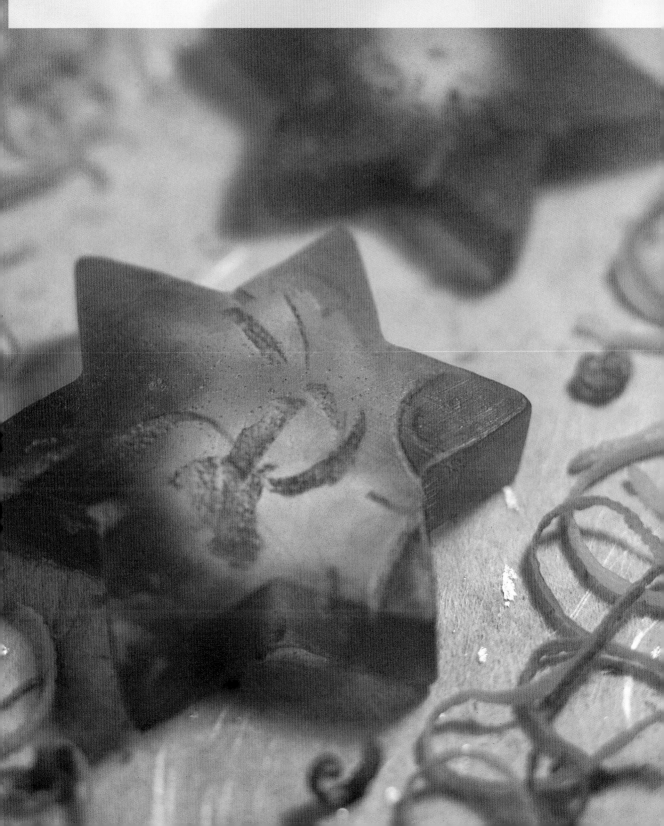

Tip: *If you prefer the clean, sharp fragrance of lemon to orange, you can make Lemon Star soaps by substituting lemon essential oil for orange, omitting the orange peel, and substituting yellow color for orange.*

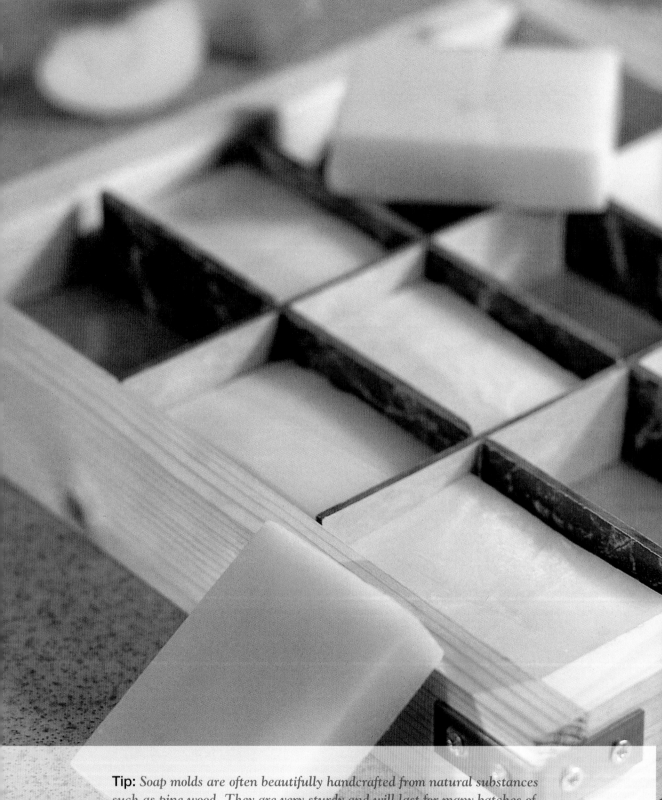

Tip: *Soap molds are often beautifully handcrafted from natural substances such as pine wood. They are very sturdy and will last for many batches of soap making.*

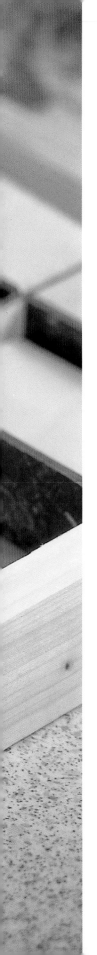

Cold-Process Vegetable Soap

Cold-process soap is what most people generally consider as "real" soap. All the other soaps you have read about earlier—and hopefully tried out!—have all included a ready-made soap base of some kind. Whether the base was liquid soap, bubble bath, grated block glycerin, or soap flakes, you still have not yet tried your hand at making soap from scratch. Now the moment has finally arrived.

One reason to try out the other soap recipes first is to develop skill and experience in working with soap. Making soap from scratch does not seem so daunting after making other kinds of soap. You will now be working with the building blocks of soap, the caustic soda (known as lye when it is dissolved in water) and base oils. The fusion of these into soap is a chemical process and is the real magic of making cold-process vegetable soap.

Basic Vegetable Soap

This is a simple soap without any additions, so you can practice this recipe a few times until you feel confident enough to add perfume, nutrients, and color. Be prepared for the odd failure; very few soap makers get it perfect on their first attempt. If your first batch or two don't work and you have to throw them away, at least you have not wasted essential oils and nutrients, which can be expensive. This basic vegetable soap is also lovely to use, and is especially suitable for people with sensitive skin, as there is no fragrance or color.

what's in it?

16 oz (455 gm) distilled water

6 oz (170 gm) of caustic soda

12 oz (340 gm) coconut oil

12 oz (340 gm) light olive oil (not extra virgin)

20 oz (567 gm) soya bean oil

how's it made?

1 Place the water in a lye- and heat-resistant container with a good pouring spout. Wearing rubber gloves and safety glasses or goggles, slowly pour the caustic soda into the water.

2 Gently stir the mixture until all the soda has dissolved, being careful to avoid splashing. The temperature of the lye will soar to well over 100°F (38°C), so leave to one side to cool.

3 Place the coconut oil, olive oil, and soya bean oil in a lye-resistant saucepan and heat gently, stirring to mix thoroughly and to evenly distribute heat. When the temperature is approximately 99°F (37°C), remove from the heat.

4 Keep measuring the temperature of both solutions, and adjust if necessary by using a water bath (see page 122). When both solutions are exactly the same temperature, ideally 97°F (36°C) (although anything between 95°F [35°C] and 100°F [38°C] should work), slowly pour the lye into the oils. You should pour slowly but steadily, stirring gently and often.

5 Once all the lye is combined with the oils, continue to stir constantly but slowly; avoid creating air bubbles. Be sure to mix thoroughly enough to incorporate the two solutions.

6 Be vigilant for signs of tracing—when the mixture turns opaque and thickens. As soon as this happens, pour the soap into greased molds. Seal the mold with plastic wrap, cover with blankets, and place in a warm, dry spot for forty-eight hours.

7 After forty-eight hours, remove the plastic wrap. You now must assess the soap. Remember to wear rubber gloves, as the soap is not yet cured and is still caustic.

8 Gently touch the surface of the soap. If it is still quite soft, leave it to sit unwrapped for another forty-eight hours. If the soap is firm to the touch, but still soft enough to leave an imprint, then unmold the soap carefully.

9 If you used one large mold, trim off any rough or uneven edges, and place on waxed paper to cure. When the soap is quite firm to the touch and pressing on it no longer leaves any imprints, it's time to cut it into individual bars. Start checking after a week.

10 If you used individual molds, once the bars are removed from the molds, place on wax paper to finish curing.

11 In both cases, you need to leave the bars of soap to finish curing in a dry, draft-free place for two to three weeks. After the final curing period, the soap should be hard, just like a commercially bought bar of soap.

12 Scrape off any surface ash that may have come out and trim the bars of soap to make them neat. The soap is now ready to use.

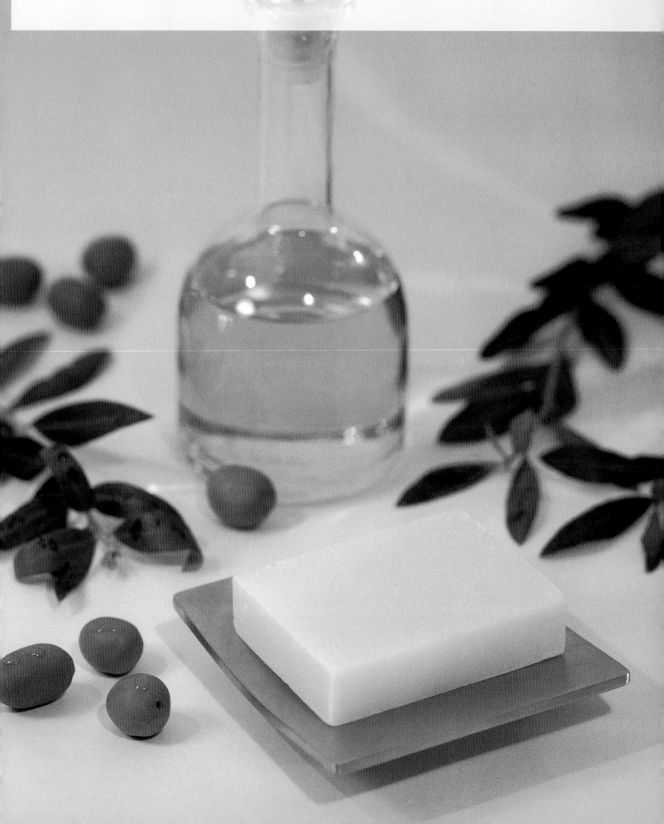

Tip: *Make sure you have plenty of time before you start, as this recipe takes more time than you might expect. Remember that all ingredients, even liquids, are measured as weight and not volume as this is the most accurate. Refer back to Basic Techniques on page 122.*

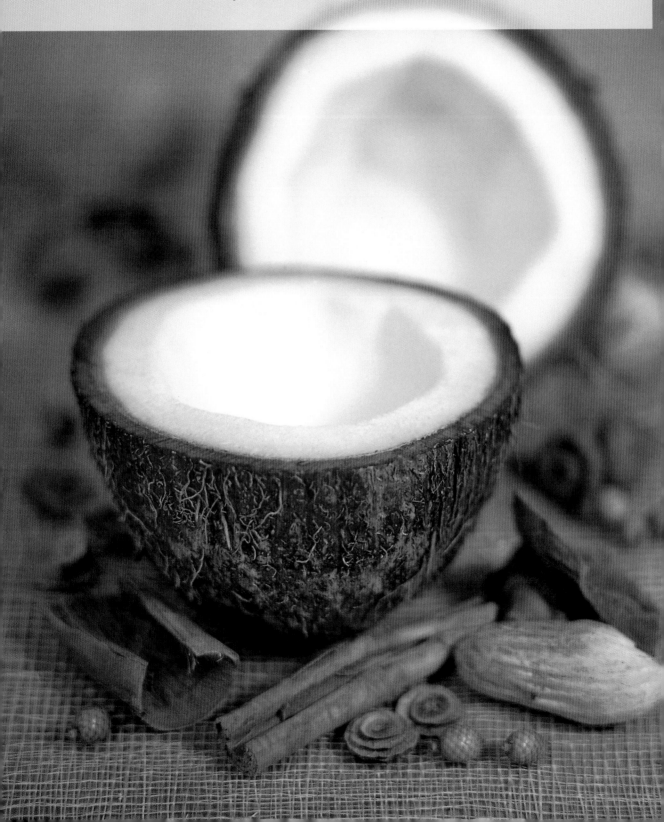

Tip: *This recipe includes essential oils, but if you prefer unscented soap, this recipe is still luxurious without any added essential oils. Simply leave out the essential oils and carry on with the next step.*

Luxury Soap

This soap contains all the best base oils and most effective nutrients used in soap making. These ingredients make Luxury Soap the best soap possible. It is kind to the skin, protecting and nourishing it, and is a real treat to use. However, the ingredients are expensive, so you probably won't want to make this soap very often. Nonetheless, you—and your friends and family if you are feeling generous!—will appreciate using these gourmet soaps.

what's in it?

16 oz (455 gm) water	8 oz (227 gm) palm oil
6 oz (170 gm) caustic soda	1½ oz (43 gm) shea butter
10½ oz (298 gm) light olive oil	15 drops sandalwood
2 oz (57 gm) apricot kernel oil	15 drops jasmine
2½ oz (71 gm) sweet almond oil	10 drops neroli
2 oz (57 gm) jojoba oil	10 drops orange
2 oz (57 gm) avocado oil	5 drops patchouli
2 oz (57 gm) kukui nut oil	5 drops chamomile
13 oz (369 gm) coconut oil	

how's it made?

1 Place the water in a lye- and heat-resistant container with a good pouring spout. Wearing rubber gloves and safety glasses or goggles, slowly pour the caustic soda into the water.

2 Gently stir the mixture until all the soda has dissolved, being careful to avoid splashing. The temperature of the lye will soar to well over 100°F (38°C), so put it to one side to cool.

3 Place all the base oils, together with the shea butter, in a lye-resistant saucepan and heat gently, stirring to mix thoroughly and to evenly distribute heat. When the temperature is approximately 82°F (28°C), remove from the heat.

4 Keep measuring the temperature of both solutions, and adjust if necessary by using a water bath (see page 122). When both solutions are exactly the same temperature, ideally 80°F (27°C), slowly pour the lye into the oils. You should pour slowly but steadily, stirring gently and often.

5 Once all the lye is combined with the oils, continue to stir constantly but slowly; avoid creating air bubbles. Be sure to mix thoroughly enough to incorporate the two solutions.

6 Be vigilant for signs of tracing—when the mixture turns opaque and thickens. As soon as this happens, drop in the essential oils and stir in thoroughly, then pour the soap into greased molds. Seal the mold with plastic wrap, cover with blankets, and place in a warm, dry spot for forty-eight hours.

7 After forty-eight hours, remove the plastic wrap. You now must assess the soap. Remember to wear rubber gloves, as the soap is not yet cured and is still caustic.

8 Gently touch the surface of the soap. If it is still quite soft, leave it to sit unwrapped for another forty-eight hours. If the soap is firm to the touch, but still soft enough to leave an imprint, then unmold the soap carefully.

9 If you used one large mold, trim off any rough or uneven edges, and place on waxed paper to cure. When the soap is quite firm to the touch and pressing no longer leaves any imprint, it's time to cut it into individual bars. Start checking after a week.

10 If you used individual molds, once the bars are removed from the molds, place on wax paper to finish curing.

11 In both cases, you need to leave the bars of soap to finish curing in a dry, draft-free place for two to three weeks. After this final curing period, the soap should now be hard, just like a commercially bought bar of soap.

12 Scrape off any surface ash that may have come out, and trim the bars of soap to make them neat. The soap is now ready to use.

Rosemary, Geranium, and Lemon

This fresh herbal and citrus smelling soap is a favorite among both sexes. Invigorating rosemary is balanced with geranium, and the addition of lemon gives a refreshing note to the blend. Cocoa butter is a rich emollient that both softens and protects the skin, making this soap a pampering indulgence.

what's in it?

16 oz (455 gm) distilled water	20 drops geranium
6 oz (170 gm) caustic soda	15 drops rosemary
12 oz (340gm) coconut oil	15 drops lemon
12 oz (340 gm) light olive oil	5 drops lavender
(not extra virgin)	5 drops basil
20 oz (565 gm) soya bean oil	5 drops frankincense
1 oz (30 gm) cocoa butter	

how's it made?

1 Follow the instructions for Basic Vegetable Soap (see page 178), adding the cocoa butter in at step 3, until just before tracing begins. Make sure you have the other ingredients close at hand.

2 As soon as the soap starts tracing, add the essential oils. Stir in thoroughly.

3 A variation on this soap is to add a few dried rose or geranium petals, which should be added at this point. This gives the soap a dappled appearance.

4 Follow the instructions for pouring into the mold and curing as you would for the Basic Vegetable Soap.

Cinnamon, Almond, and Honey

This earthy brown soap is laden with organic ground cinnamon, which also makes this soap gently exfoliating. The honey and almond oil add richness to the soap, and both are hydrating and moisturizing for the skin. The spice oils are reminiscent of soft winds over tropical islands. Their fragrance is balanced with a hint of sweetness from the honey and the voluptuous ylang ylang.

what's in it?

16 oz (455 gm) distilled water	2 tsp (10 ml) organic ground
6 oz (170 gm) caustic soda	cinnamon
12 oz (340 gm) coconut oil	15 drops cinnamon
12 oz (340 gm) light olive oil	10 drops clove
(not extra virgin)	10 drops black pepper
20 oz (565 gm) soya bean oil	10 drops grapefruit
1 oz (30 gm) sweet almond oil	10 drops ylang ylang
1 oz (30 gm) warmed honey	5 drops frankincense

how's it made?

1 Follow the instructions for Basic Vegetable Soap (see page 178), until just before tracing begins. Make sure you have the other ingredients close at hand.

2 As soon as the soap starts tracing, add the almond oil, warmed honey, cinnamon, and essential oils. Stir in thoroughly.

3 Alternatively, leave the cinnamon until you have thoroughly mixed in the other ingredients, and simply swirl in at the end to create a marbled effect.

4 Follow the instructions for pouring into the mold and curing as you would for the Basic Vegetable Soap.

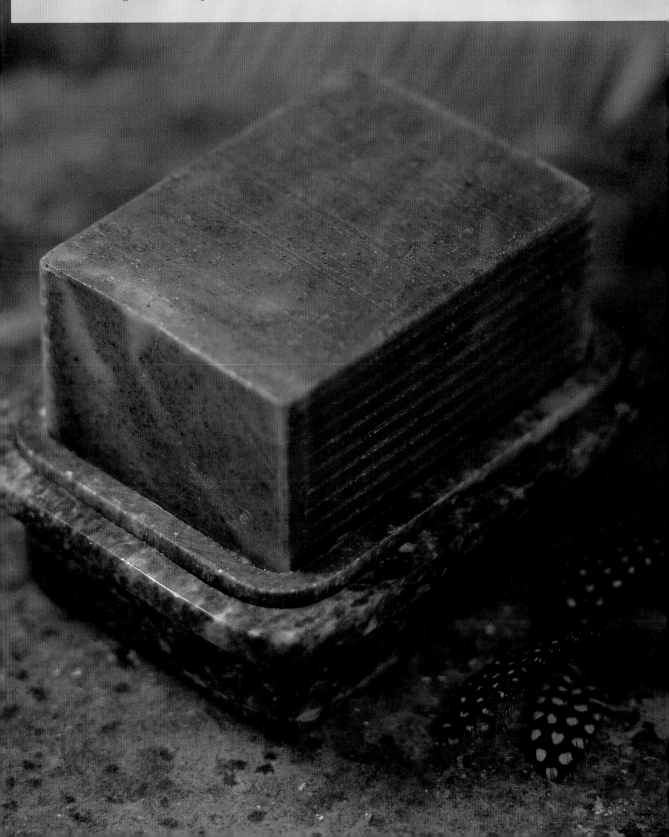

Tip: *You can use less cinnamon for a more subtle effect. Adding it at the end and briefly swirling it in gives a marbled mosaic finish, which is very attractive. Experiment with both quantity of cinnamon and technique of adding it to the soap.*

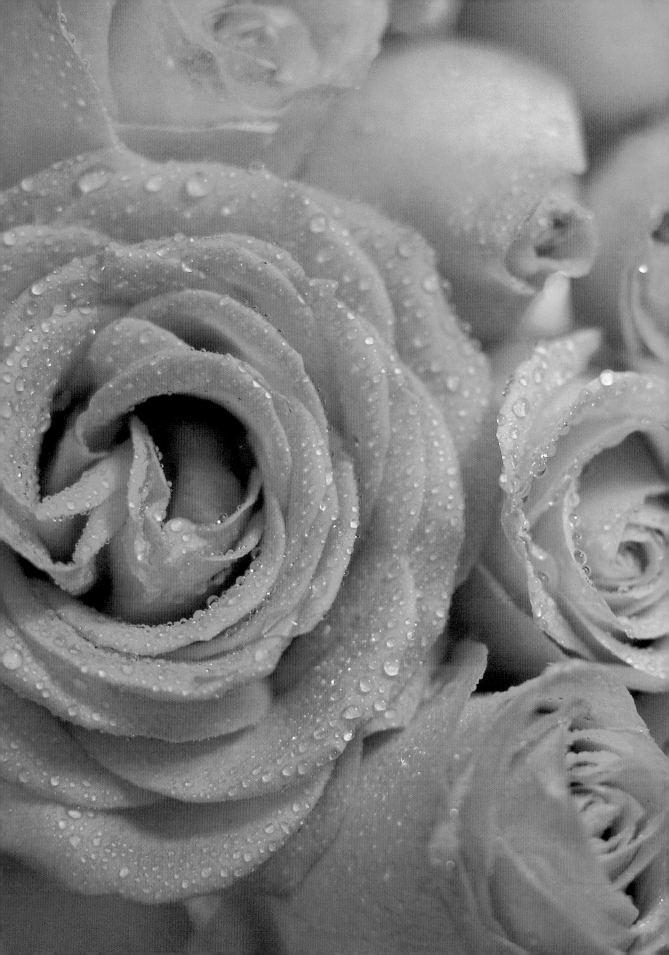

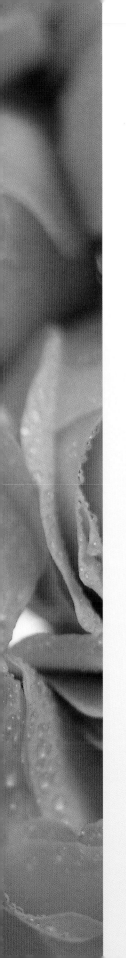

Chapter 13

Natural Scents

The Art of Perfuming

The art of perfuming has been with us for many centuries, and the ancient civilizations were surprisingly adept at creating scents. There are perfume jars and bottles dating as far back as 3500 BC. Traditionally, perfumes were used for other purposes in addition to personal scents. The most important use of perfume was to please the gods, and perfume in the form of incense was burnt daily so the aromatic smoke would ascend to the heavens.

Aromatic woods, gums, and resins such as frankincense and myrrh were used in the embalming of bodies in ancient Egypt. The ancient Indian medicinal system, Ayurveda, used, and still uses today, sandalwood and saffron in medicinal remedies. Herbs and spices are used throughout the world to scent food and make it appetizing. The overwhelming focus of the perfume industry however is in the arena of personal scents.

The center of the fragrance industry is in Grasse, France. Huge fields of lavender and other flowers and herbs are grown to provide the raw materials for distilling essential oils, one of the prime ingredients of perfumes. Factories for distillation and the creation of perfume are scattered throughout the area. Famous perfume recipes are highly guarded secrets, and each perfume house employs a top "nose"—a highly trained individual who can distinguish between the thousands of different fragrances.

Commercial perfumes are highly complex blends of essential oils, animal derivatives such as musk and ambergris, and high-proof alcohol. It takes a long time to create a fragrance, and hundreds of different ingredients in differing proportions will be tried before one definitive recipe is decided upon. Perfumes are classified into "families," each with a specific character. The most familiar of these are: floral, green, chypre, citrus, aldehydic, oriental, and oceanic. For example, the popular sophisticated modern perfume Opium belongs in the oriental family.

Making your own scents need not be a daunting prospect if you follow a few simple guidelines. All the perfumes in this book use only essential oils, preferably organic, and no animal products. Some perfumes are oil based, and others use alcohol diluted with flower waters. Both these types of perfume are easy to blend. Each perfume needs to have a top note, a middle note, and a base note, to create harmony, like in music. This makes a balanced fragrance that has both an immediate impact and a lasting quality.

Perfuming is an art, and wearing perfume is a personal choice. So after following a few of the following recipes, you could create your own personalized scents. These will reflect your personal creativity, character, and mood. It is intensely satisfying to make and wear your own personal fragrances and it is a creative form of self expression.

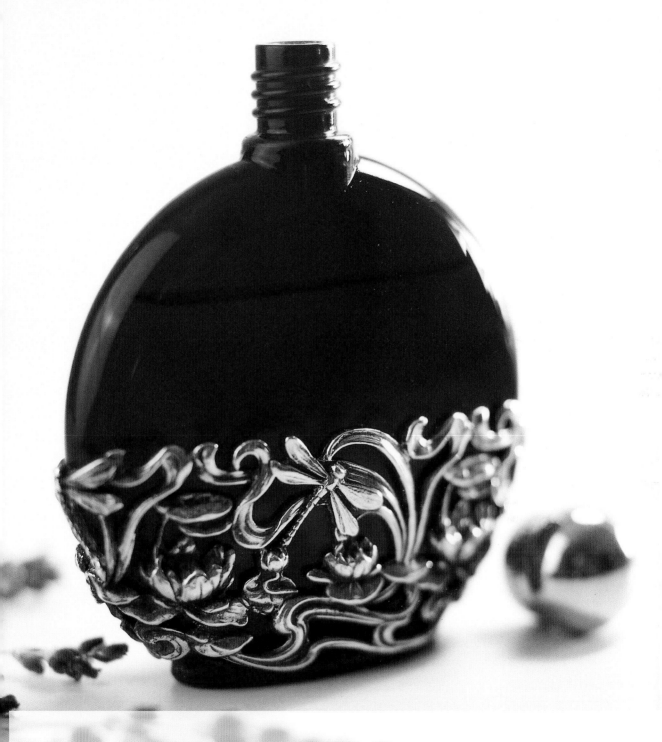

"Making scents at home is experimenting with and creating customized fragrances—sprays, essences, perfume oils, colognes, and waters—that blend with and reflect personal emotions, moods, and lifestyles."
–Catherine Bardey, *fashion stylist and author*

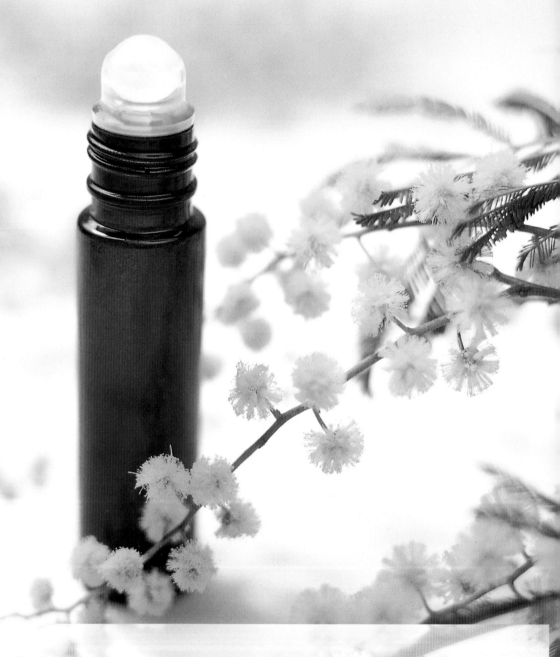

Tip: *Oil-based perfumes don't last as long as the alcohol-based perfumes. The rollette bottles are ½ fl oz (10 ml) size and can easily be used up in less than six months. After this time, the perfume will be past its best and may start to degenerate.*

Perfume Roll-ons

Perfume roll-ons are oil-based perfumes dispensed from small roll-on bottles. These are glass bottles with a rollette plastic ball insert; they are easily purchased from one of the suppliers listed on pages 222–223. Perfume roll-ons are both simple to make and convenient to carry in a handbag, so you can freshen up your perfume throughout the day and evening. The four perfume recipes in this section comprise two floral fragrances, one citrus, and one oriental.

Floral is the largest of the perfume families. Floral perfumes suit feminine, delicate personalities, and are especially suited for wearing in the daytime and in the spring and summer. Citrus perfumes are breezy, light, and fresh. They suit the youthful and are exuberantly feminine. They are suited to daytime and casual evening wear. Oriental fragrances are heavy, mysterious, and seductive. They suit the mature, sophisticated personality and are best worn in the evening.

Provence Floral

This delightfully feminine fragrance is influenced by the classic floral perfumes such as L'Air du Temps, Joy, and Chanel No. 22. The light floral essential oils, blended subtly with a little citrus, gives a top note that is light, fresh, and floral. The middle note is deeper, with the calm aroma of chamomile bringing a slightly bitter green note. Hints of frankincense and sandalwood provide a long lasting bottom note, which stabilizes the overall fragrance.

what's in it?

1 tbsp (10 ml) sweet almond oil
10 drops rose
10 drops lavender
10 drops neroli
4 drops mimosa
3 drops geranium
4 drops chamomile
3 drops bergamot
3 drops frankincense
3 drops sandalwood

how's it made?

1 Fill a small glass jar with a lid with 1 tablespoon (10 ml) of sweet almond oil.

2 Line up the bottles of essential oils. If you don't have every one of the essential oils mentioned in the recipe, don't worry. Add the number of drops of the missing oil to one of the other oils, or simply leave them out.

3 Carefully drop in the essential oils, one by one. Shake the jar vigorously, and leave for fifteen minutes for the oils to adjust themselves in the blend.

4 Pour the perfume into a ½ fl oz (10 ml) glass rollette bottle, using a funnel if necessary. Push the roll-on ball in firmly, and screw on the cap. The perfume is now ready to use, but will improve subtly over the next few days.

Fresh and Fruity

This lively, breezy fragrance is ideal for the younger woman, and makes a good first perfume. Neither too heavy nor serious, the delicate fragrance is clean, refreshing, and clear. The citrus oils are complemented by light floral and woody tones. The merest hint of an herbal tone gives a slight green middle note, which balances the citrus top notes.

what's in it?

1 tbsp (10 ml) sweet almond oil

7 drops orange

7 drops mandarin

10 drops bergamot

7 drops petitgrain

5 drops neroli

5 drops rosewood

3 drops clary sage

2 drops ambrette seed

4 drops ylang ylang

Romantic Rose

Roses and rose perfumes have always been among the most popular of fragrances since ancient times. There are quite a few different types of roses grown to produce rose oil, and they all differ slightly. The color of the essential oil ranges from greenish orange to brownish red, and each rose oil will have a slightly different aroma, although it will be unmistakably rose. This perfume uses a few different types of rose oil to give an intense rose fragrance. Rose oil is expensive, so this perfume is a luxurious treat, but if you love roses, this is a wonderful perfume.

what's in it?

1 tbsp (10 ml) sweet almond oil

15 drops rose otto

15 drops rose absolute

10 drops rose geranium

3 drops bergamot

4 drops patchouli

3 drops palmarosa

how're they made?

1 Fill a small glass jar with a lid with 1 table-spoon (10 ml) of sweet almond oil.

2 Line up the bottles of essential oils. If you don't have every one of the essential oils mentioned in the recipes, don't worry. For Romantic Rose, however, you do need to have at least one of the rose oils, but you can adjust the number of drops of each oil according to what you have.

3 Carefully drop in the essential oils, one by one. Shake the jar vigorously, and leave for fifteen minutes for the oils to adjust in the blend.

4 Pour the perfume into a ½ fl oz (10 ml) glass rollette bottle, using a funnel if necessary. Push the roll-on ball in firmly, and screw on the cap. The perfume is now ready to use, but will improve subtly over the next few days.

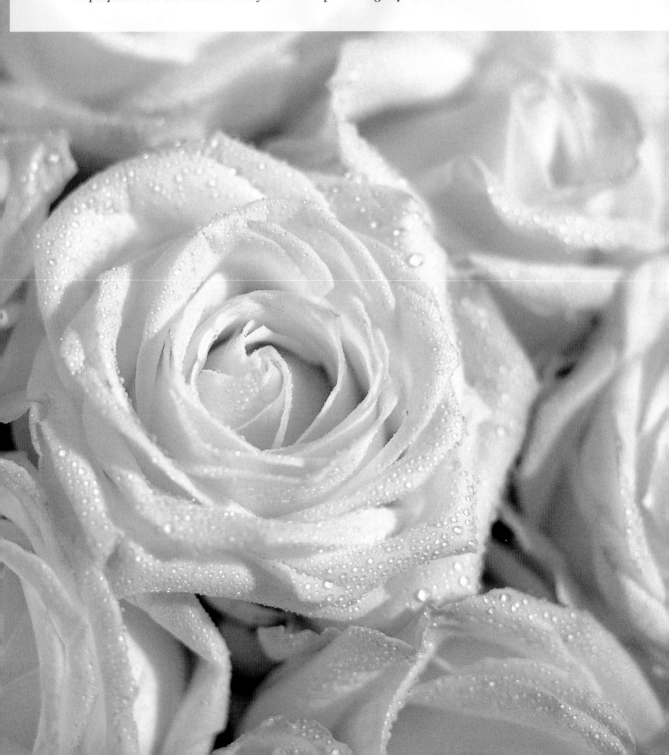

Did You Know? *Rose oil is probably the most valued essential oil in the perfume industry. Approximately three-quarters of all top-class, quality perfumes on the market today include a percentage of rose oil.*

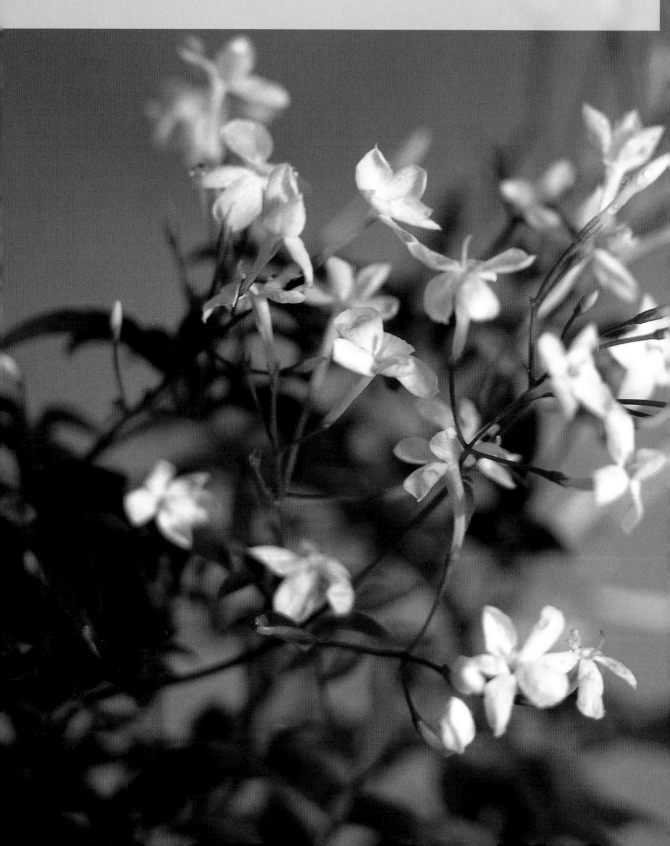

Did You Know? *The distillation process from which essential oils are derived was probably discovered accidentally by Avicenna, the great Arab physician, during an alchemical experiment with roses.*

Amorous Dreams

This is a mysterious perfume ideal for a romantic evening or a late night party. Deep, sweet, floral top notes mingle with woody, spicy middle notes and long lasting earthy, resinous undertones. Patchouli became popular in the 1960s, and was often worn as a perfume on its own. Here, it is a lot more subtle, and blended with floral, citrus, spice, and woody oils to create a delightful mystical fragrance.

what's in it?

1 tbsp (10 ml) sweet almond oil

7 drops patchouli

7 drops jasmine

10 drops bergamot

7 drops rose

3 drops vanilla

2 drops myrrh

5 drops sandalwood

3 drops clove

2 drops violet leaf

4 drops nutmeg

how's it made?

1 Fill a small glass jar with a lid with 1 tablespoon (10 ml) of sweet almond oil.

2 Line up the bottles of essential oils. If you don't have every one of the essential oils mentioned in the recipe, don't worry. Add the number of drops of the missing oil to one of the other oils, or simply leave them out.

3 Carefully drop in the essential oils, one by one. Shake the jar vigorously, and leave for fifteen minutes for the oils to adjust themselves in the blend.

4 Pour the perfume into a ½ fl oz (10 ml) glass rollette bottle, using a funnel if necessary. Push the roll-on ball in firmly, and screw on the cap. The perfume is now ready to use, but will improve subtly over the next few days.

Splash Colognes

Colognes are light, fresh fragrances that are all derived from the traditional eau de cologne. The original eau de cologne was made in the early part of the eighteenth century by Johann-Maria Farina, an Italian living in Cologne, Germany. His cologne quickly became famous for its cooling, deodorant, and refreshing qualities, and by the end of the eighteenth century there were many different versions available.

Commercially made colognes use perfume-grade ethyl alcohol as the base, but this is impossible to purchase in small quantities. For the recipes below, use the highest proof vodka you can find. This is diluted slightly with a flower water, which adds to the overall fragrance, and has a less drying effect on the skin than neat alcohol. As they are not highly concentrated perfumes, you can splash these colognes on generously.

Citrus Cologne

This recipe is a simple version of the original eau de cologne, and has a familiar classic fragrance. The perfume is clean and fresh, with citrus top notes, a light floral middle note, and a green herbal base note.

what's in it?

4 tbsp (50 ml) high proof vodka

40 drops bergamot

25 drops lemon

10 drops neroli

15 drops lavender

10 drops petitgrain

7 drops rosemary

3 drops thyme

2 tbsp (25 ml) orange flower water

how's it made?

1 Fill a dark glass bottle (which can hold 4 fl oz [100 ml] of liquid) with the high proof vodka.

2 Carefully drop in the essential oils, one by one. Put on the bottle cap and shake vigorously for a few minutes to thoroughly dissolve the essential oils.

3 Top off with the flower water, and shake again. A small amount of essential oil may separate out and float on the top, so before using the cologne, remember to shake the bottle first each time.

4 Let the cologne stand for a week or two before using it. This allows the cologne to mature and the perfume to settle.

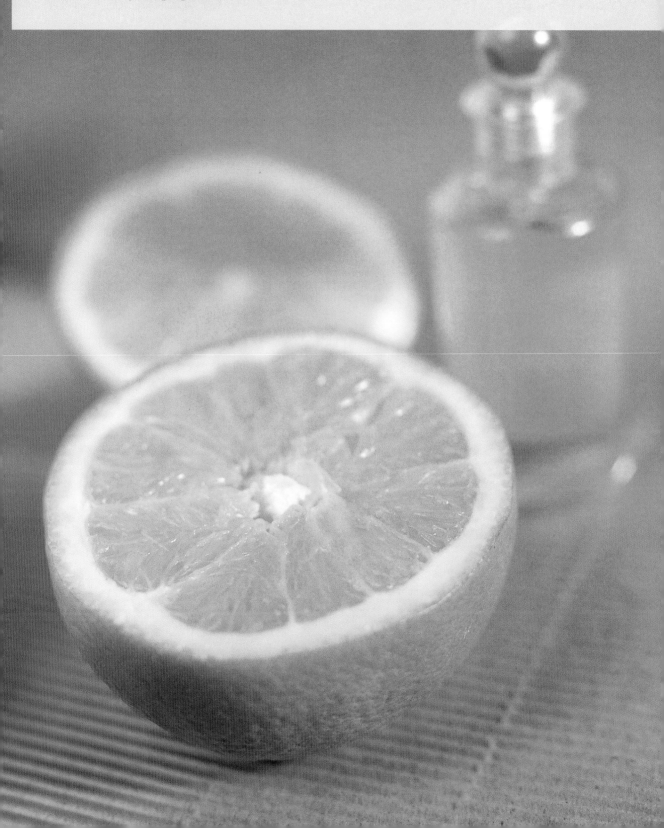

Did You Know? *Napoleon was notoriously fastidious about personal hygiene, and used lots of eau de cologne. He even took it along and used it during his military campaigns.*

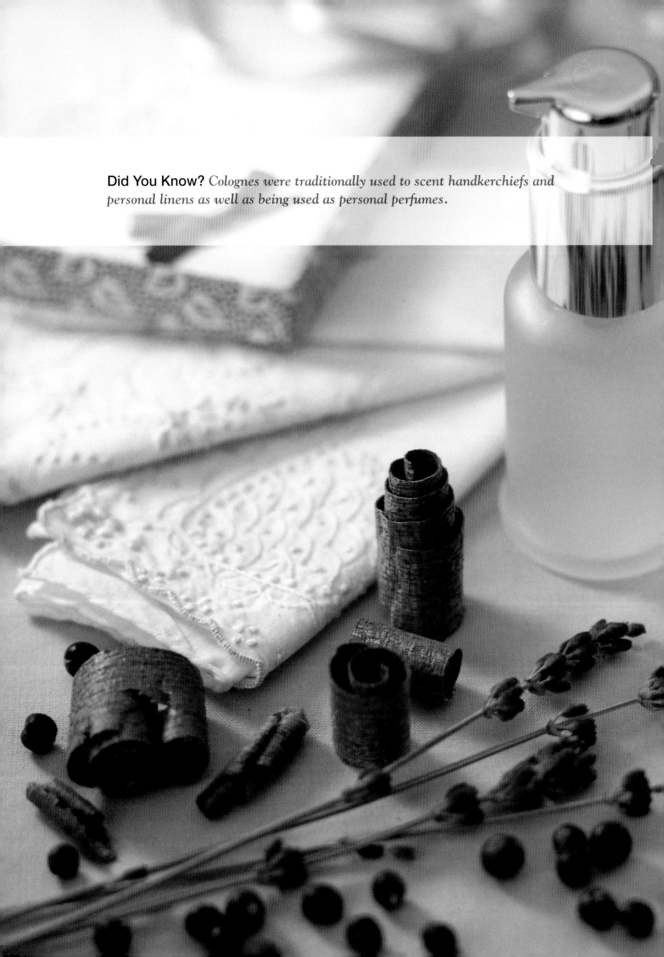

Did You Know? *Colognes were traditionally used to scent handkerchiefs and personal linens as well as being used as personal perfumes.*

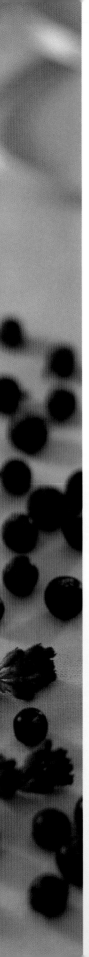

Deep and Mysterious

The traditional eau de cologne is suitable for both women and men. Deep and Mysterious has a green, woody, spicy fragrance that might be described as masculine, and is particularly suited to men, though not exclusively of course! Perfume is a personal choice, and you should wear what perfumes you like, whether they are described as suitable for you or not.

what's in it?
4 tbsp (50 ml) high proof vodka
20 drops vetiver
10 drops frankincense
15 drops lemon
5 drops black pepper
15 drops neroli
25 drops cedarwood
10 drops juniper
5 drops marjoram
5 drops clary sage
2 tbsp (25 ml) lavender flower water

Sweet and Gentle

This is a lovely, delicate, feminine cologne with hints of citrus and a honeyed sweet undertone. Particularly well suited to wear on days when you feel in need of some emotional support, this cologne surrounds you in a haze of comforting scent.

what's in it?
4 tbsp (50 ml) high proof vodka
20 drops linden blossom
10 drops bergamot
20 drops neroli
15 drops lavender
15 drops mandarin
5 drops jasmine
5 drops ambrette seed
10 drops rosewood
10 drops geranium
2 tbsp (25 ml) rose flower water

how're they made?

1 Fill a dark glass bottle (which can hold 4 fl oz [100 ml] of liquid) with the high proof vodka.

2 Carefully drop in the essential oils, one by one. Put on the bottle cap and shake vigorously for a few minutes to thoroughly dissolve the essential oils.

3 Top off with the flower water, and shake again. A small amount of essential oil may separate out and float on the top, so before using the cologne, remember to shake the bottle first each time.

4 Let the cologne stand for a week or two before using it. This allows the cologne to mature and the perfume to settle.

Manly Musk

This is another masculine fragrance with a distinctive musky note. Although musk itself is derived from animals, there are essential oils that give a musky fragrance. Nutmeg in particular is used in the perfume industry for its musklike aroma. Clove is another spice oil that has been used in perfumes extensively, and was one of the main ingredients used by the early Arab perfume makers.

what's in it?
4 tbsp (50 ml) high proof vodka
20 drops sandalwood
10 drops frankincense
20 drops nutmeg
15 drops clove
15 drops petitgrain
5 drops jasmine
10 drops vetiver
5 drops holy basil
10 drops clary sage
2 tbsp (25 ml) linden flower water

how's it made?

1 Fill a dark glass bottle (which can hold 4 fl oz [100 ml] of liquid) with the high proof vodka.

2 Carefully drop in the essential oils, one by one. Put on the bottle cap and shake vigorously for a few minutes to thoroughly dissolve the essential oils.

3 Top off with the flower water, and shake again. A small amount of essential oil may separate out and float on the top, so before using the cologne, remember to shake the bottle first each time.

4 Let the cologne stand for a week or two before using it. This allows the cologne to mature and the perfume to settle.

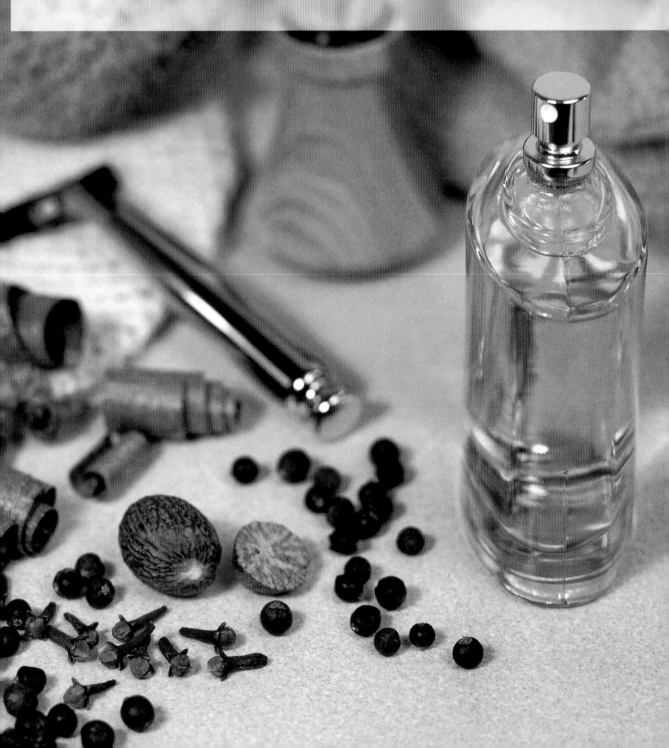

Did You Know? *Perfumes have not always been approved of. The Greek philosopher Plato considered perfumes immoral and likely to lead to licentious behavior.*

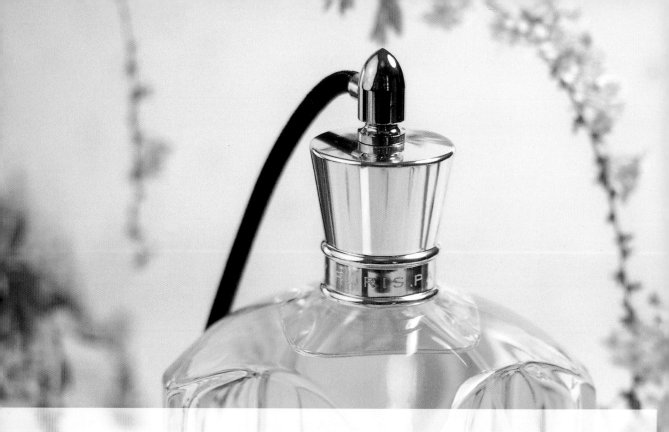

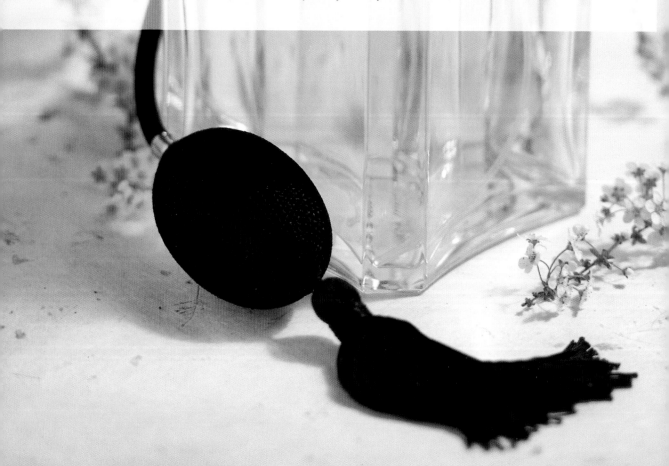

Tip: *Try carrying this body spray with you when you are traveling on a hot, sticky day. Remembering to shut your eyes first, spray the Summer Breezes over your face to cool down and refresh yourself.*

Body Sprays

How we apply perfume varies according to fashion. For instance, in ancient Rome, slave girls would dance with aromatic cones on their heads. The perfume was blended into a base of fat, so that when the girls became hot through dancing, the fat melted and the perfumed oil would drip down over their hair and bodies. In the modern world, perfumed body sprays are fashionable. These are dilute aromatic toilet waters that can be sprayed all over the body to give an overall fragrant effect. This provides an alternative to the more selective application of concentrated perfume to the pulse points behind the ears, inside of the wrists, and base of the throat.

The following body sprays are based on flower waters and essential oils that make natural plant-based perfume sprays. Many of the perfumed sprays commercially available are based on synthetic compounds and chemicals, which can cause allergies. These natural body sprays are much kinder to your skin and smell wonderful too.

Summer Breezes

On a hot summer's day, a cooling, perfumed body spray is a real treat to use. This perfume has hints of fresh mown hay and apples from the chamomile, together with green herbal and sweet floral notes. A tiny trace of citrus and spice gives the perfume a clean, sharp tang.

what's in it?

2 tsp (10 ml) high proof vodka
20 drops chamomile
10 drops linden blossom
10 drops geranium
10 drops clary sage
10 drops lavender
5 drops bergamot
5 drops coriander
5 drops neroli
6 tbsp (90 ml) rose water

how's it made?

1 Fill a 3 fl oz (100 ml) or 4 fl oz (125 ml) glass bottle—with a spray attachment—with the high proof vodka.

2 Carefully drop in the essential oils, one by one. Shake the bottle vigorously to dissolve the essential oils.

3 Top off with the rose water, and shake to mix thoroughly.

4 Let the perfume stand for a few days to settle and mature. Shake the bottle before using the perfume each time, as a few drops of essential oil may not be fully dissolved.

Lavender Calmer

Lavender is well loved for the calming effect it has on the emotions. Here it is blended with ylang ylang, which is deeply relaxing and sensuous, and neroli, which is a sweet smelling nerve tonic. Hints of citrus give a light top note to this sweet, floral calming perfume.

what's in it?

2 tsp (10 ml) high proof vodka

20 drops lavender

20 drops neroli

10 drops ylang ylang

10 drops lemon

5 drops bergamot

5 drops rosewood

5 drops palmarosa

6 tbsp (90 ml) cornflower water

how's it made?

1 Fill a 3 fl oz (100 ml) or 4 fl oz (125 ml) glass bottle—with a spray attachment—with the high proof vodka.

2 Carefully drop in the essential oils, one by one. Shake the bottle vigorously to dissolve the essential oils.

3 Top off with the cornflower water, and shake to mix thoroughly.

4 Let the perfume stand for a few days to settle and mature. Shake the bottle before using the perfume each time, as a few drops of essential oil may not be fully dissolved.

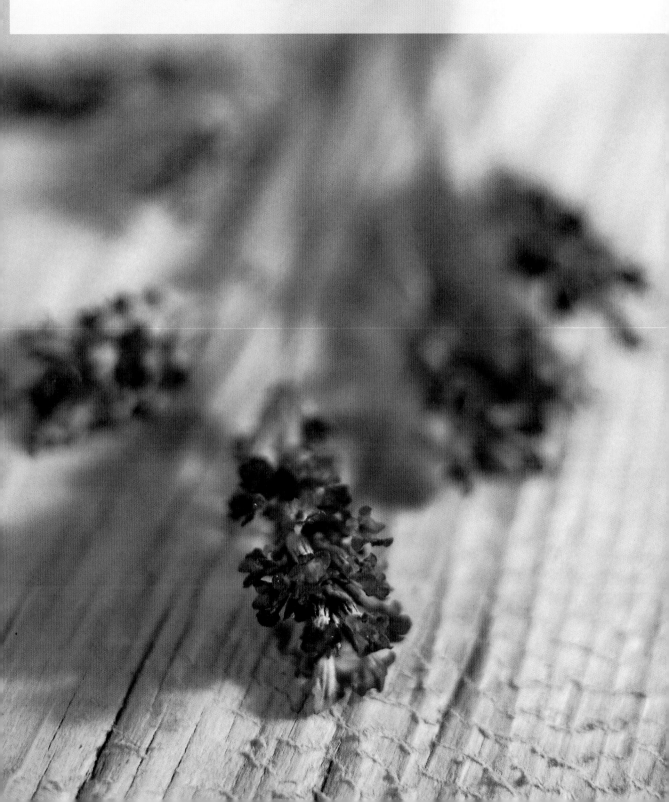

Did You Know? *The Lavender Calmer recipe uses cornflower water, which is one of the more unusual flower waters. It has a lovely, fresh, calming scent. However, if you don't have cornflower water, then this recipe is also good using rose or lavender flower waters instead.*

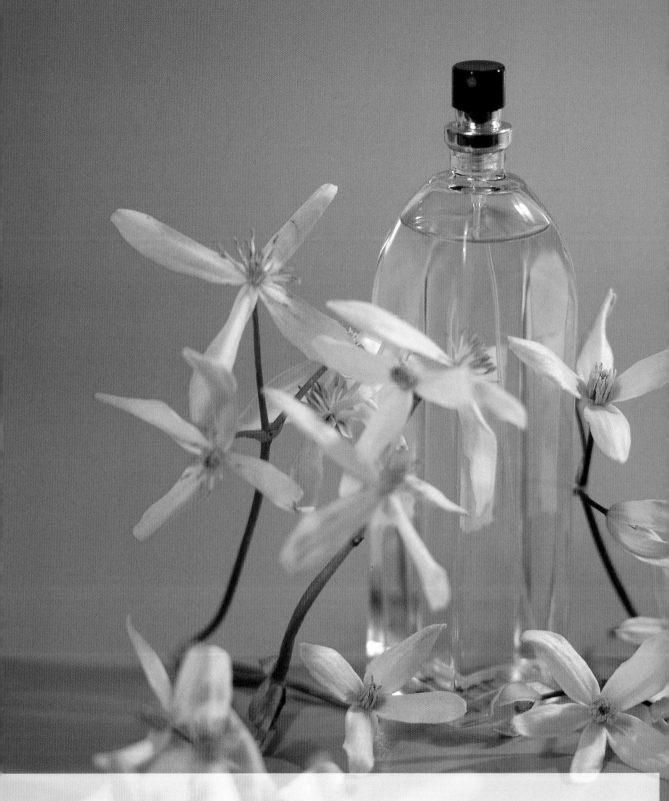

Did You Know? *Bergamot is a citrus fruit, closely related to the orange, and is generally regarded as the finest of the citrus fruits. Bergamot is featured in about forty percent of commercial perfumes.*

Orange Flower Blossom

This sweet, orange floral perfume reunites all the produce of the orange tree. Petitgrain is derived from the wood of the orange tree, orange is from the fruit, and neroli is from the orange flower blossom. The overall effect is a clean, sweet orange perfume that is full of laughter and smiles.

what's in it?

2 tsp (10 ml) high proof vodka
20 drops orange
20 drops neroli
20 drops petitgrain
10 drops bergamot
5 drops mandarin
6 tbsp (90 ml) orange flower water

how's it made?

1 Fill a 3 fl oz (100 ml) or 4 fl oz (125 ml) glass bottle—with a spray attachment—with the high proof vodka.

2 Carefully drop in the essential oils, one by one. Shake the bottle vigorously to dissolve the essential oils.

3 Top off with the orange flower water, and shake to mix thoroughly.

4 Let the perfume stand for a few days to settle and mature. Shake the bottle before using the perfume each time, as a few drops of essential oil may not be fully dissolved.

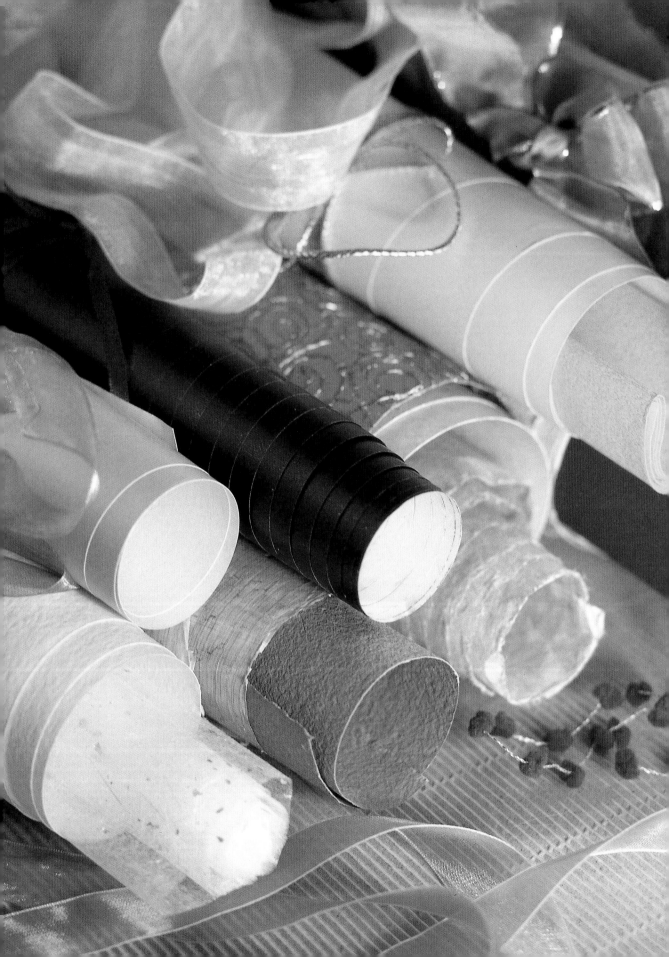

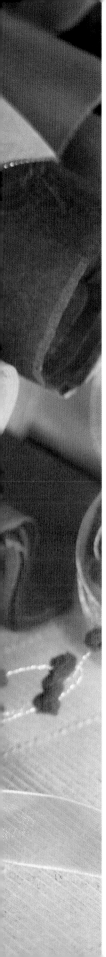

Chapter 14

Presenting
Soaps and Scents

Packaging and Decoration

Once you have made a batch or two of hand-crafted soap, it's time to think of how to package it. Because the soaps are natural, plant based, and use organic ingredients, it is appropriate for the packaging to reflect this. There are some beautiful natural packaging materials available. These include recycled corrugated cardboard, raffia, handmade papers, wicker baskets, and other natural packaging materials.

There are no hard and fast rules for packaging soaps, although using a breathable material is generally considered best for the soap. You can experiment with fabrics, dried banana leaves, and woods, as well as the materials mentioned above. Fragrant soaps made with essential oils should be wrapped as soon as possible after the curing process or drying time. The packaging acts a barrier against the air, so the scent is retained longer.

You may want to consider decorating your soaps before you package them. Although soaps made with spices, dried flowers, herbs, poppy seeds, or oats already have color and texture, you can add further detail. Plain soaps can be transformed by decoration. Some of the soap recipes suggest pushing a dried rosebud into the soap before it hardens. An alternative is to use melted paraffin wax—or candle wax—to affix a dried flower to the top of the soap after it has hardened. You could also affix an almond, vanilla pod, coffee bean, or section of cinnamon stick to indicate what ingredients went into the soap.

Another way to decorate your soap is to make an imprint. This should be done when the soap is firm, but not quite hard, in the middle of the curing or drying process. For an antique feel, use an old wax sealing stamp, the kind used to seal letters. You can find other stamps in kitchen stores among the cookie cutters and cake decorating utensils. These offer an imaginative alternative. Whatever implement you use, grease it first with a little vegetable oil so you make a clear, clean imprint, and so that it does not stick.

Scents are easier to pack than soaps, as they have already been made in or poured into a bottle. You can use ornamental glass bottles rather than plain glass bottles, so the perfumes are presented attractively. There is a wide range of ornamental glass bottles available, with etched glass, colored glass, stained glass, and decorated glass all having a different appeal. A range of bottles can be displayed on a dressing table or shelf for a dramatic effect.

If you are making a gift of a perfume bottle, then you can wrap the bottle in colored tissue paper to protect the fragile glass, and place this in a decorative box. Glass bottles are the traditional containers for scents, but if you want a historical feel, you can look for stone or porcelain bottles. These can make stunning gifts. Natural-colored sandstone bottles from India are particularly effective for a natural, organic look. Delicate porcelain bottles, sometimes available with spray attachments, offer a refined, sophisticated feel.

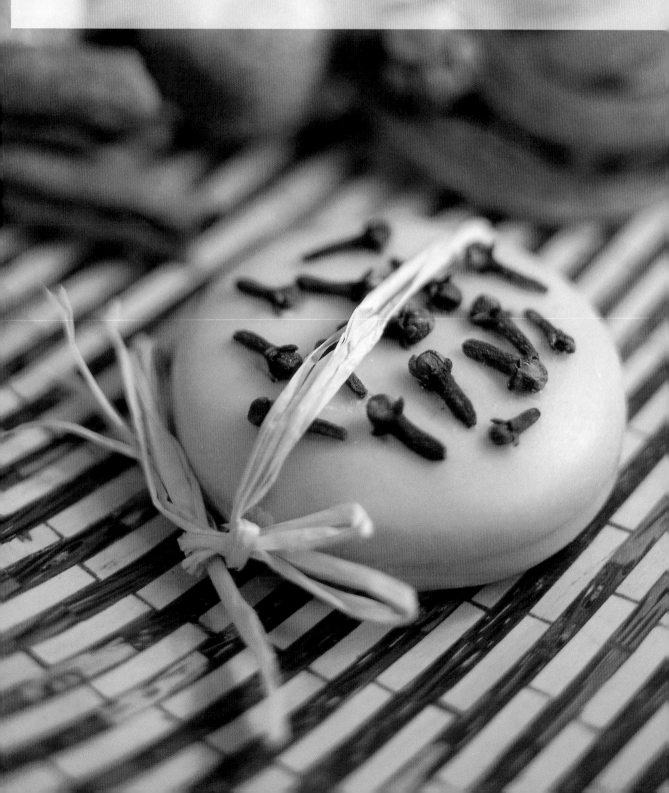

"The packaging material you select will depend on what look you want to give your soap."

—Catherine Bardey, *fashion stylist and author*

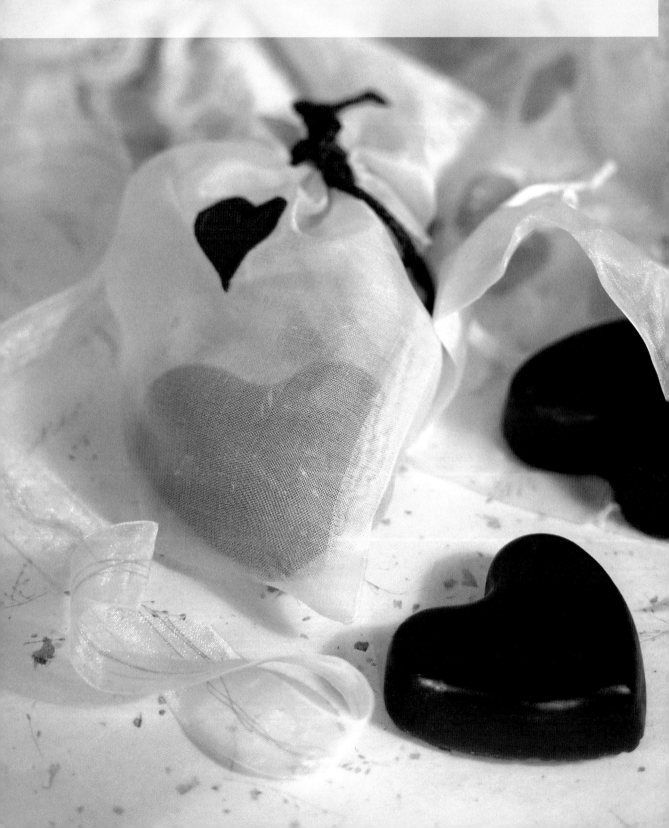

Tip: *Patterned translucent material or wrapping paper make particularly effective wrapping for glycerin soaps.*

Gift Wrapping

Wrapping your soaps in imaginative ways can make them look really professional and pretty. Here are some ideas for gift wrapping your soaps.

Choose a square of fabric according to what look you'd like to give the soap. Coarse, natural fabrics such as hessian or hemp give an organic feel and look, while silk and satin offer a more sophisticated look. Wrap the soap in the fabric just as you would a parcel. Tie a natural, organic cloth with raffia or brown string, and tie a silk or satin wrapped soap with a pretty ribbon.

Cut a strip of decorative or handmade paper that is half the length of the soap bar you want to wrap. Wrap round the middle of the soap so the two ends are exposed. To personalize the soap, affix a handmade label to the center of the decorative wrap. This can either describe the type of soap or it can be a personal design.

Make a drawstring pouch from natural or decorative fabric. Lace makes a particularly interesting pouch, and reveals the perfume and appearance of the soap. Create the drawstring by sewing a strip of fabric over a ribbon or cord at one end of the piece of fabric, leaving enough space so the cord can be drawn tight.

Wrap the soap bar in a simple square of plain white muslin. Choose some decorative dried flowers or herbs on stems that reflect the ingredients used in the soap. Use raffia or ribbon to tie a decorative bow around the muslin, and tie up the flower stems with the ribbon, so the flowers create an attractive bunch on the top of the wrapped soap.

You can make a strand of small soaps, wash balls, or bath bombs. Take a rectangular sheet of fabric and lay it on a flat surface. Allowing for a two inch (5 cm) border, place the individual soaps along the long edge of the fabric with a two inch (5 cm) space in between each soap. Carefully fold the fabric over the soaps and roll them up into a strand. Tie the ends and the spaces between the soaps with ribbon, string, or raffia. Finally, you can trim the ends of the fabric with pinking shears for added decorative effect.

Make a pretty lace effect with a paper doily. Place a bar of soap in the center, and gently gather up the edges to a bunch at the top. Tie up the bundle with a strip of lace. You can include the stems of a few dried rosebuds or other dried flowers in the lace, so the flower buds fall decoratively around the doily parcel.

Boxes and Ribbons

Once you've wrapped your soaps, you can pack them into boxes for a practical finishing touch. Although the soaps are quite hard, they can still be damaged even when wrapped. If you want to mail soaps as a gift to someone, putting them in a box first will protect them. However, the boxes can still be decorative and you can tie these with ribbons to make a beautiful gift. Here are some ideas for packing your soaps decoratively using boxes and ribbons.

As the quotation suggests, you can find small wooden crates and fill these with soaps. Try including both wrapped and unwrapped soaps nestled among shredded paper. You can make a bed of dried flowers and nestle a selection of unwrapped bars of soap for an organic look. For a more professional look, wrap soap bars in different colored tissue paper and alternate these in the crate. If the crate has slats, you can weave some raffia or ribbons in and out of the slats for added effect.

Natural, organic soaps can make a beautiful arrangement in a small wicker box or basket. Try placing dried baby pinecones and ornamental grasses in the bottom of a wicker basket and placing soap on the top. Wrap a sheet of cellophane around the arrangement, and glue the ends together underneath the basket. Take several strands of different colored raffia or ribbons and plait or weave them together, and then tie this over the top.

You can make a box using a sheet of corrugated cardboard. Place soap in the middle of a sheet of corrugated cardboard. With a sharp knife, gently score lines across the surface of the cardboard where you want to make the folds. The cardboard will then fold snugly to make a neat box. Take a long, wide velvet ribbon, and tie into a decorative bow. Carefully cut the long ends of the ribbon into strips, and tie a single rosebud at the end of half of the strips of ribbon for a stylish effect.

Take a cardboard box and half fill with potpourri. Place one or more soaps in among the potpourri and scatter more of the dried flowers and leaves on the top, so the soaps are half hidden. Seal the box, and tie a pretty ribbon around the box to

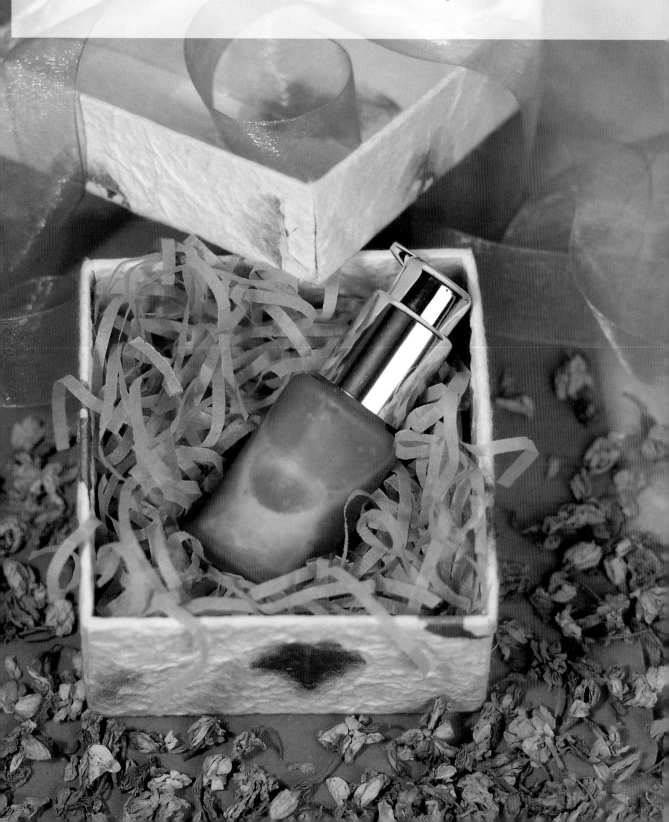

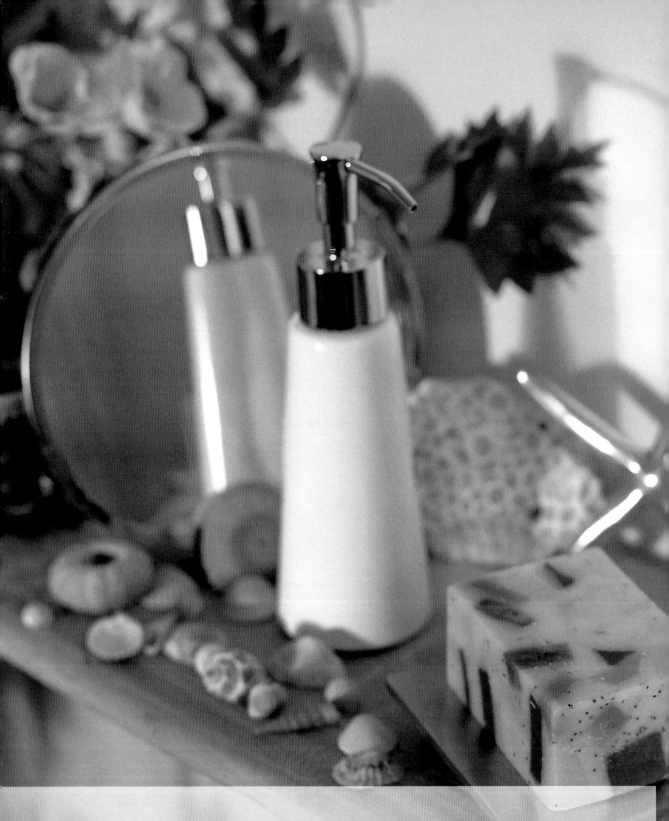

Tip: *A selection of scattered sea shells mingled amongst your soaps looks very attractive on a bathroom shelf.*

Displaying Your Soaps and Scents

Once you've made a range of soaps and scents, you will want to display all your hard efforts beautifully. In this way you can really appreciate how lovely your soaps and scents are. You've already read some ideas about how to decorate, wrap, and present your soaps and scents as gifts for others. Now you can try out some ideas on displaying soaps and scents in your home for yourself and your family.

Displaying your homemade scents is easy because they are already in pretty bottles, and look enchanting wherever you put them. One particularly attractive display is to line up a few bottles of your favorite scents in front of your dressing table mirror. The reflection of the bottles adds to the effect of the bottles themselves, and can make quite a dramatic sight.

Although your scent bottles should not be exposed to light, you can make an entrancing display by using empty scent bottles. You can also fill them with water to give the illusion of full scent bottles. Choose a small window with a window sill that has some direct sun for at least part of the day. Take a variety of crystals and attach fine silk or plastic thread to each one. Hang at different levels in the window, making sure a few hang right down to the window sill. Line up your bottles of scent among the hanging crystals. When the sun shines, you will have a magical scene of dancing reflections from the crystals and bottles.

Find a pretty soap dish to display your soaps on the bathroom basin and kitchen sink. You can also use other dishes and containers for a stunning effect. Try small white ceramic bowls, glass and stainless steel dishes, more often found among tableware. Japanese and Chinese stores have plenty of pretty ceramic dishes that can double up as attractive soap dishes.

For a really dramatic effect on the bathroom basin, use a thick slab of colored glass, or a trimmed piece of industrial metal. If you find a suitable but rough piece, most large hardware stores will be able to trim off any sharp edges for you. A tiny section of a wrought iron fence or gate makes an effective soap dish that also drains well.

A bathroom shelf, or freestanding bathroom unit, can take a display of soaps. In this way you can enjoy looking at them before you use them. They also give off a light delicate fragrance. Try making a tower of different soaps, with a couple of larger bars at the base, and building up to a small bar or wash ball on the top.

Handcrafted soaps mingled in with towels and linens on a bathroom shelf looks attractive, and the soaps also impart a hint of their fragrance to the linen. You can alternate along the shelf so you have a pile of towels next to a stack of soaps with perhaps a vase of dried flowers in the middle before another stack of soap and pile of towels.

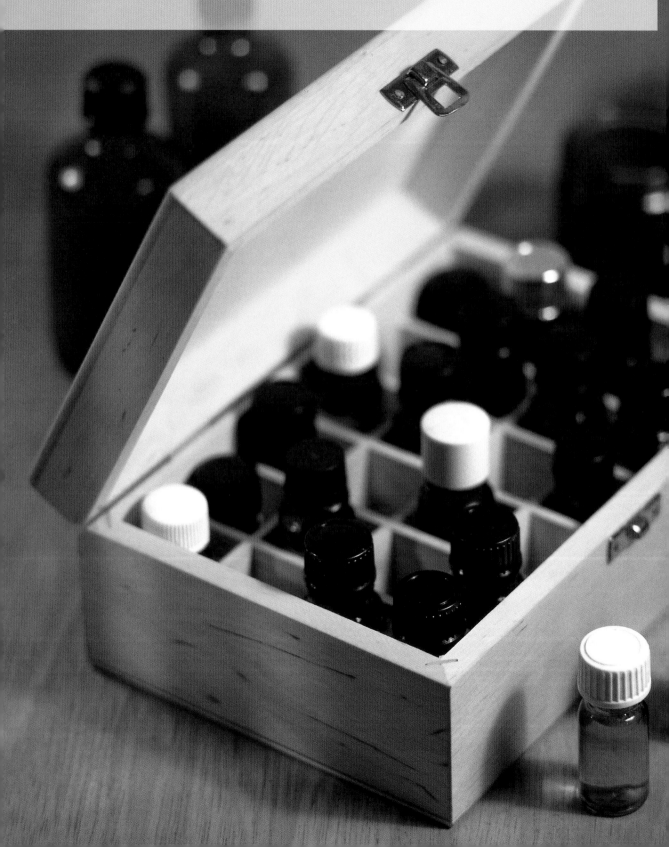

Resources

Buying and storing all your soap and perfume-making ingredients properly is fundamentally important to the overall process of making soaps and scents. The suppliers listed in the directory on pages 222–223 give you a range of suppliers of all the ingredients and equipment you will need to successfully make soaps and scents. Below are tips on buying and storing your ingredients properly, and also tips on storing your soaps and scents once you've made them.

- All ingredients are best bought fresh. Although the various ingredients for soaps and scents have differing shelf lives, it is a good habit to buy your ingredients only as you need them.

- Only buy sufficient quantities for your immediate requirements. Even though buying in bulk may be cheaper, unless you use it up quickly it could prove a false savings.

- Store your ingredients in a cool, dark, dry place away from drafts, light, damp, and heat. This will help prolong shelf life.

- Make sure you store your bottles of essential oils upright, in a cool dark place.

- Fresh ingredients such as fruits should be as fresh as possible, especially organic produce.

- If you have used half a bag of soap flakes, laundry starch, or similar dry product, make sure you reseal the bag well and remove all air. Or you could transfer the remainder into a airtight plastic container.

- Color bases of ground spices in oil will keep for a couple of months in an airtight, dark glass jar.

- If you think something has spoiled because it has discolored or changed texture, throw it away and buy new supplies. Using old ingredients could affect how a recipe turns out, and you don't want to waste other ingredients.

- Handcrafted soaps will last between six months and a year if you store them away from dust and excess light once they have fully dried out or cured. A helpful tip is to give away extra soaps as you make them, so you are not left with a cupboard full.

- Homemade scents based on oil will last up to six months. Scents based on alcohol will last a lot longer, as alcohol is a natural preservative. Scents based on flower waters are best used up within three months.

Troubleshooting

Here are some of the common problems that arise from cold-process soap making, together with a few hints on how to avoid them.

Tracing does not occur

Tracing can require a lot of patience, as it may still happen well after the time it's supposed to. Don't give up until you are quite sure the mixture is not going to trace, or after twenty-four hours. The probable reasons why tracing did not occur are: too much water or not enough lye, temperature was too high or too low, stirring the mixture ineffectually or too slowly. Next time ensure you measure all ingredients accurately and the temperature of fats and lye precisely.

The soap mixture is grainy

This is an aesthetic problem only, and the soap is safe to use. Grainy soap is caused by too high or too low temperatures, or by not stirring briskly or regularly enough.

The soap is soft and spongy

It is unlikely these bars will harden enough to use, so throw them away. Soft soap is caused by not using enough lye.

The soap is hard and brittle

You must throw these bars away as they are too alkaline for the skin. Hard soap is caused by using too much lye.

Air bubbles in the soap

Check that the bubbles only contain air. If there is liquid in the bubbles, you will have to throw the soap away, because the liquid will be mostly lye. If the bubbles are only air, the soap is fine to use. Air bubbles are caused by stirring too briskly (whipping or beating the mixture) or stirring for too long before pouring into the mold.

The soap mixture separates

Here you end up with a layer of hard soap underneath an oily liquid top layer. This soap must be thrown away. Separation is caused by insufficient stirring, too much lye, being poured into the mold too soon, or once poured the soap cooled too quickly.

Soap is marbled with white streaks

Make sure there are no chunks of slippery, solid lye. If they are just streaks then the soap is fine to use. Streaking is caused by uneven stirring, the temperature at which the lye and fats were mixed was too cold, or the soap was stirred for too long after adding the essential oils.

Curdling

The soap looks a bit like cottage cheese, or has small, pearly lumps forming at the bottom of the pan. The soap should be thrown away. Curdling is caused by inaccurate measurements or incorrect temperatures, irregular stirring, or cooling too quickly.

Soap has hard white chunks after hardening

Throw this soap away as the chunks are lye and the soap is too caustic to use. This is caused by using too much lye or stirring was too slow or ineffective.

Excessive soda ash on top of the cured soap

A small amount of soda ash is expected from the curing process. This is harmless and can easily be trimmed off. If, however, there is a lot and you have to cut deep into the soap to remove it, then the soap is too alkaline and must be thrown away. Excessive soda ash is caused by using too much lye.

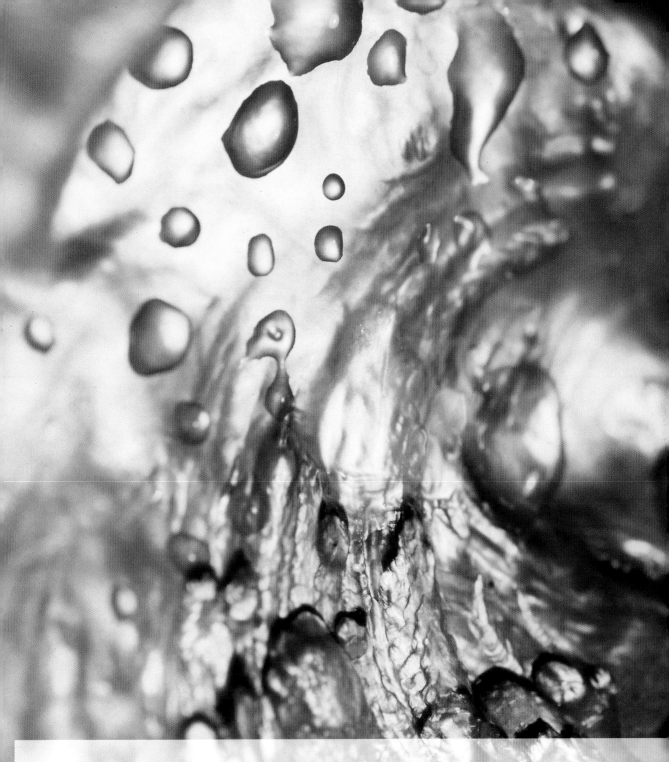

Tip: *Take careful, detailed notes each time you make soap, including descriptions of each stage of the soap making. If something isn't quite perfect the first time, then you can make minor adjustments to quantities and procedures to improve things next time around.*

Glossary of Ingredients

Almond Oil (more precisely sweet almond oil):
A base oil and a nutrient that can be used in all different types of home-made cosmetics and soap. Also, a prime ingredient in making skin creams, and ideal as a base for roll-on perfumes.

Avocado Oil:
A nutrient oil high in vitamins A, D, and E and fatty acids. Contains healing properties and is easily absorbed by the skin. Used to enrich skin creams and soaps with its excellent moisturizing qualities.

Beeswax:
A natural by-product of honey, available unrefined as a yellow block or refined as white pellets. Used in skin creams and lip balms.

Block Glycerin:
Used to make glycerin soaps.

Caustic Soda:
Also known as lye when in solution. Chemical name is sodium hydroxide. It is the alkaline or base used in cold-process soap making.

Cocoa Butter:
A rich nutrient good for softening and protecting the skin. Used to enrich skin creams, lotions, and soaps.

Coconut Oil:
A solid oil at room temperature that melts on contact with the skin. Used primarily in making coconut oil hand creams. Also, a prime base oil in cold-process soap making with unparalleled lathering and moisturizing properties.

Essential Oils:
Distilled from herbs, flowers, woods, resins, and citrus fruits. Used to enrich and perfume toners, creams, lotions, shampoos, and conditioners.

Flower Waters:
Including rose water, orange flower water, cornflower water and linden blossom water. Flower waters are also know as hydrolats. Used in skin toners, eye washes, deodorants, face creams, and skin lotions.

Honey:
Natural healing nutrient used in face packs and lip balms.

Jojoba Oil:
Actually a liquid wax. Excellent moisturizing qualities. Helps skin retain normal sebum levels and it is used to enrich skin creams and lotions.

Kukui Nut Oil:
An excellent moisturizing nutrient. Has been shown to help heal skin conditions such as acne, eczema, psoriasis, and sunburned skin. Used in creams and lotions.

Liquid Glycerin:
A syrupy, clear liquid that is good for moisturizing and healing dry skin. A nutrient used to enrich skin creams.

Monoi de Tahiti:
A soft, waxy block made from coconut oil and perfumed with gardenia flowers. Used to enrich and perfume creams and lotions.

Oat Plant Milk:
Made with natural lipids and vegetable proteins. Very mild and gentle on the skin and hair. Used to enrich creams, lotions, and hair conditioners.

Rosehip Granules:
Ground dried rosehips with a slightly grainy texture. Used in body scrubs as an exfoliant; gives a pinky-peach color to soaps and gives a slightly grainy texture.

Rosehip Oil:

The best available is Rosa Mosquetta. It is high in essential fatty acids and gamma linolenic acid and helps regenerate the skin. A healing nutrient used to enrich creams and lotions.

Shea Butter:

Also known as Karite nut butter. Excellent skin moisturizing qualities especially healing for dry, damaged, and irritated skin. A valuable nutrient in creams, lotions, and soaps.

Soya Bean Oil:

A prime base oil for cold-process soap making. Contributes bulk, mildness, and a stable lather. Best used in combination with other oils and nutrients that have good skin moisturizing qualities.

Spices and Herbs:

Ground spices and herbs are used to color soaps naturally. The most common include alkanet root, turmeric, cinnamon, and paprika.

Witch Hazel
(actually distilled witch hazel):

Distilled from the herb hamamelis virginiana, witch hazel is a commonly used astringent. Used in skin toners, aftershaves, and deodorants.

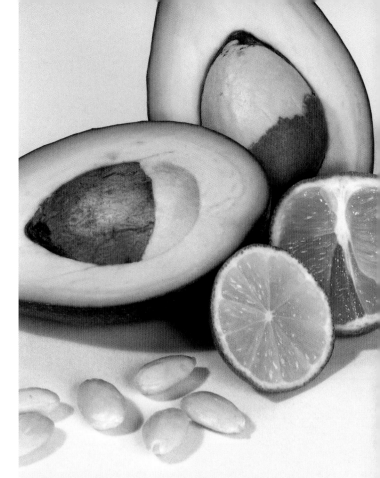

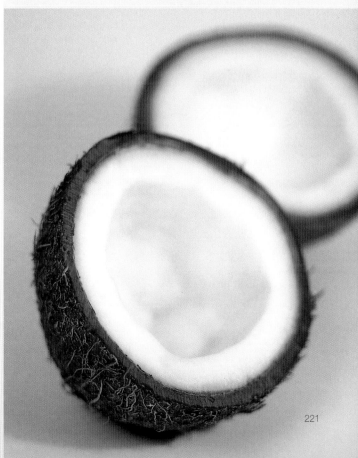

221

Suppliers

Angel Earth
1633 Scheffer Avenue
St Paul, MN 55116 USA
(651) 698-3601

Aphrodisia Products Inc.
264 Bleeker Street
New York, NY 10014 USA
(212) 989-6440

**Aquarius Aromatherapy
& Soap**
PO Box 2971
Sumas, WA 98295-2971 USA
info@aquariusaroma-soap.com

Butterbur & Sage
Aroma house
7, Tessa Road
Reading
Berkshire RG18HH UK
+44 (0) 118 9505100
butterburandsage@btinternet.com

The Essence of Life
7106 NDCBU
Taos, NM 87571 USA
(505) 758 7941
essence@taos.net.com

Essential Oil Company
8225 7th Southeast Avenue
Portland, OR 97207 USA
orders@essentialoil.com

Essentially Oils
8–10 Mount Farm, Junction Road
Churchill, Chipping Norton
Oxfordshire, OX7 6NP UK
+44 (0) 1608 659544
sales@essentiallyoils.com
www.essentiallyoils.com

Fragrant Earth Co Ltd
Orchard Court
Magdalene Street
Glastonbury BA6 9EW UK
+44 (0)1458 831216
all-enquiries@fragrant-earth.com

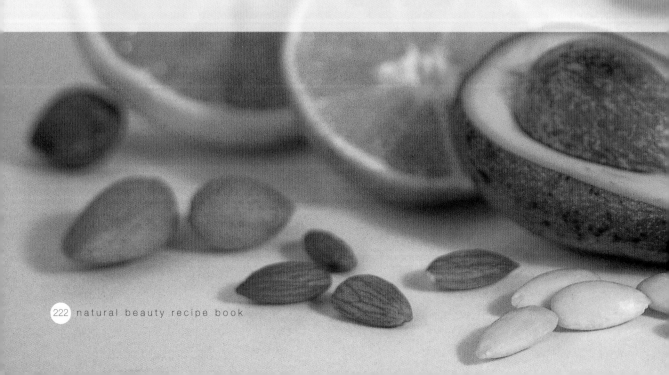

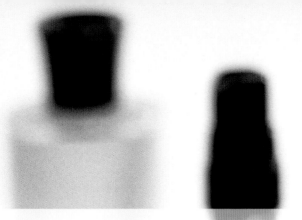

G. Baldwin & Co
171/173 Walworth Road
London SE17 1RW UK
+44 (0) 207 703 5550
sales@baldwins.co.uk
www.baldwins.co.uk

Janca's Jojoba Oil & Seed Co
550 W. Baseline Rd #102–302
Mesa, AZ 85210 USA
(480) 497-9494
www.jancas.com

Pourette
P.O. Box 70469
Seattle, Washington 98127 USA
(206) 789-3188
www.pourette.com

Prima Fleur Botanicals Inc
1525 E. Francisco Blvd Suite 16
San Rafael, CA 94901 USA
(414) 455 0957
info@primafleur.com

Sunfeather Natural Soap Company
1551 Highway 72
Potsdam, NY 13676 USA
(315) 265-3648
www.sunsoap.com

Woodspirits UK
Unit 42
New Lydenburg Industrial Estate
New Lyndenburg Street
London SE7 8NE UK
+44 (0)20 8293 4949
woodspiritsuk@compuserve.com

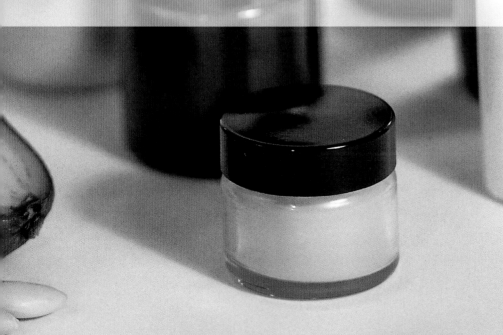

Acknowledgments

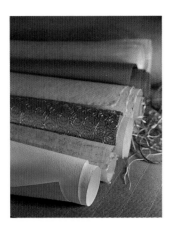

I would like to thank Robin Bath, Toby Matthews, Angie Patchell, and Winnie Prentiss for their talented assistance in bringing this book to fruition. I would also like to give a special thanks to the models, Alice Pennefather and Caroline Grealis.

I would also like to thank my partner, Robert Beer, for his loving support throughout the writing of this book, and for willingly trying out many of the different homemade cosmetics.

Thanks are also due to Chantek Mottershaw and Lotte Rose for tips and ideas on making face creams.

Nicki at Woodspirits UK provided valuable tips and support during my soap making, and supplied a few additional soaps for the photographs in this book. Nicki offers a range of beautiful handcrafted soaps (see page 223).

I would also like to thank the following UK businesses for the kind provision of materials for the photography:

4 my way of life, 13–15 Jerdan Place, Fulham, London SW6 1BE
The Chelsea Gardener, 125 Sydney Street, London SW3 6NR
Cologne & Cotton Ltd., 791 Fulham Road, London S26 5HD
Damask, 3–4 Broxholme House, New Kings Road, London S26 4AA
Paperchase, 213 Tottenham Court Road, London W1T 7PS
pH Factor, 183 New Kings Road, London SW6 4SW
toute-bagai, 160 Wandsworth Bridge Road, London S26 2UH
Sasha Waddell, 269 Wandsworth Bridge Road, London SW6 2TX
Sue Walker, 166 Wandsworth Bridge Road, London SW6 2UH